PETS IN PRACTICE

TRUDE MOSTUE

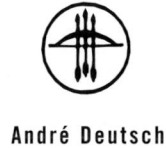

André Deutsch

Acknowledgements
The author would like to thank all the animals and the people who inspired her to write this book.
Special thanks to Lisa Strickland, Colston Cutler and Dennis Taylor

Picture credits
Ardea: pages 6, 11, 14, 22, 27, 50, 59, 71(l), 124 John Daniels, 71(r) J-P Ferrero,
94, 102, 106 John Mason; FLPA: 19 D. Dalcon, 90 Silvestris, 133 Foto Natura,
137, 140 Gerard Lacz; Don Last: 73; John Meredith: Cover pictures, 4, 30, 34, 46, 54, 82, 112 (all);
Trude Mostue: 63, 66, 79, 86, 116, 129

First published by André Deutsch Ltd
76 Dean Street
London W1V 5HA
www.vci.co.uk

Text copyright © Trude Mostue 2000
Editor: Valerie Porter

The right of Trude Mostue to be identified as the author of this book has been asserted by her
in accordance with the Copyright, Designs and Patents Act 1988. All rights reserved.
This book is sold subject to the condition that it may not be reproduced, stored in a retrieval
system or transmitted in any form or by any means, electronic, mechanical, photocopying,
recording or otherwise without the publisher's prior consent.
CIP data for this title is available from the British Library

ISBN
0-233-99781-4

Design and Editorial
designsection, Frome, Somerset

Reprographics by Radstock Reproductions
Midsomer Norton, Bath

Printed and bound in the UK by
Butler & Tanner Limited
Frome and London

CONTENTS

INTRODUCTION 4

CHAPTER 1
PETS BEHAVING BADLY 6

CHAPTER 2
EMERGENCIES 34

CHAPTER 3
BREEDS AND BREEDING – OR NOT 54

CHAPTER 4
PREVENTION – PROBLEMS THAT CAN BE AVOIDED 82

CHAPTER 5
KEEPING FIT 112

INDEX 142
USEFUL ADDRESSES 144

INTRODUCTION

I was born in Norway on a cold, wintry day. I was an ugly, screaming baby and very demanding. I grew up with my sisters, Lene and Hilde, living beside a lovely lake full of fish and ducks. We acquired a cocker spaniel when I was five years old and she spent most of her time swimming in the lake, pursuing her lifelong ambition of catching one of those ducks. We also had cats that produced lots of kittens and spent most of their time trying to eradicate the lake's rodent population.

I suppose I was first inspired to become an 'animal doctor' when my cat used to bring me my patients. Too often they were headless, or bodiless, and my mum tried to tell me that the prognosis was hopeless. Eventually, having spent my childhood trying to repair the cats' hunting victims, I began to realise that cats are extremely efficient hunters and that my patients would not survive. So, as a 10-year-old, I promised myself that I would dedicate my life to saving animals. My quest had begun.

A few years later I met a vet for the first time in my life. Despite him putting our dog to sleep and telling me that being a vet meant washing your hands a lot and having your arm up a cow's bottom, I set out to pass all the exams I needed to get into vet school. I passed my last A-level in 1987 and then decided it was time to check out if the vet was right.

For the next three years I gained a wide range of practical experience. I was herdswoman to 125 Norwegian Red dairy cattle near Oslo; I worked in a research centre, studying pigs' semen; and then I spent a year as a combination of receptionist, assistant veterinary nurse, cleaner and general handywoman in a small-animal practice in Oslo. Finally I was accepted at Bristol University to study veterinary science. In Norway there was a need to educate far more vets each year than we had the capacity to teach, and so they encouraged us to study in Britain.

TRUDE MOSTUE + Pets in Practice

Despite knowing that my English was poor (well, I could say useful things like, 'Where can I trim my moustache, please?'), I decided to pack my bags with a lot of enthusiasm, stubbornness, determination and an English dictionary.

Between my third and fourth year I escaped back to Norway to become a milkmaid for 400 goats in the beautiful fjord country. I was a real Heidi for two months, milking goats and making cheese for tourists. Ready to face the last two years of studying, I returned to the UK to finish my time at vet school. In my final year I met my first BBC film crew and the rest is history. I wept, laughed and swotted my way through that final year and, as you might know, I eventually passed, crying my eyes out in front of a BBC camera crew. It had taken six long years and a lot of tears, guts and doggedness but I had passed my finals.

I quickly found a job in Bristol, where I stayed for two years. In between working there I also spent some time in Africa working with big game – an opportunity not to be missed. My new interest in the larger, more exotic species stimulated me to apply for my second job in a veterinary practice in Somerset, which let me alternate between chasing hamsters in the surgery and chasing lions and elephants at Longleat Safari Park.

Recently I took the next big step in my veterinary career: I have just set up my own practice in Bristol with my fellow Norwegian vet, Maria Lowe.

In the meantime, I have been lucky enough to look for polar bears in Canada and wildlife in the United States as part of various BBC television series. As I have been followed by a BBC camera crew for three years, from 'Vets School' and 'Vets in Practice' to 'Vets in the Wild' and 'Vets to the Rescue', it feels as if most of my life has been on public view; in fact, it feels as if something is missing when the cameras are not there in the background. And if you are wondering whether the tears were worth it over the last few years, I would very definitely say yes!

Finally comes this book. I want to share with you stories of some of the animals I have treated – some of them with happy endings, some not, some of them funny, some of them sad, but all of the stories full of information for owners of all kinds of pets. My experience with the animals and their owners has been a rich and varied one and I would like to make you a present of that experience.

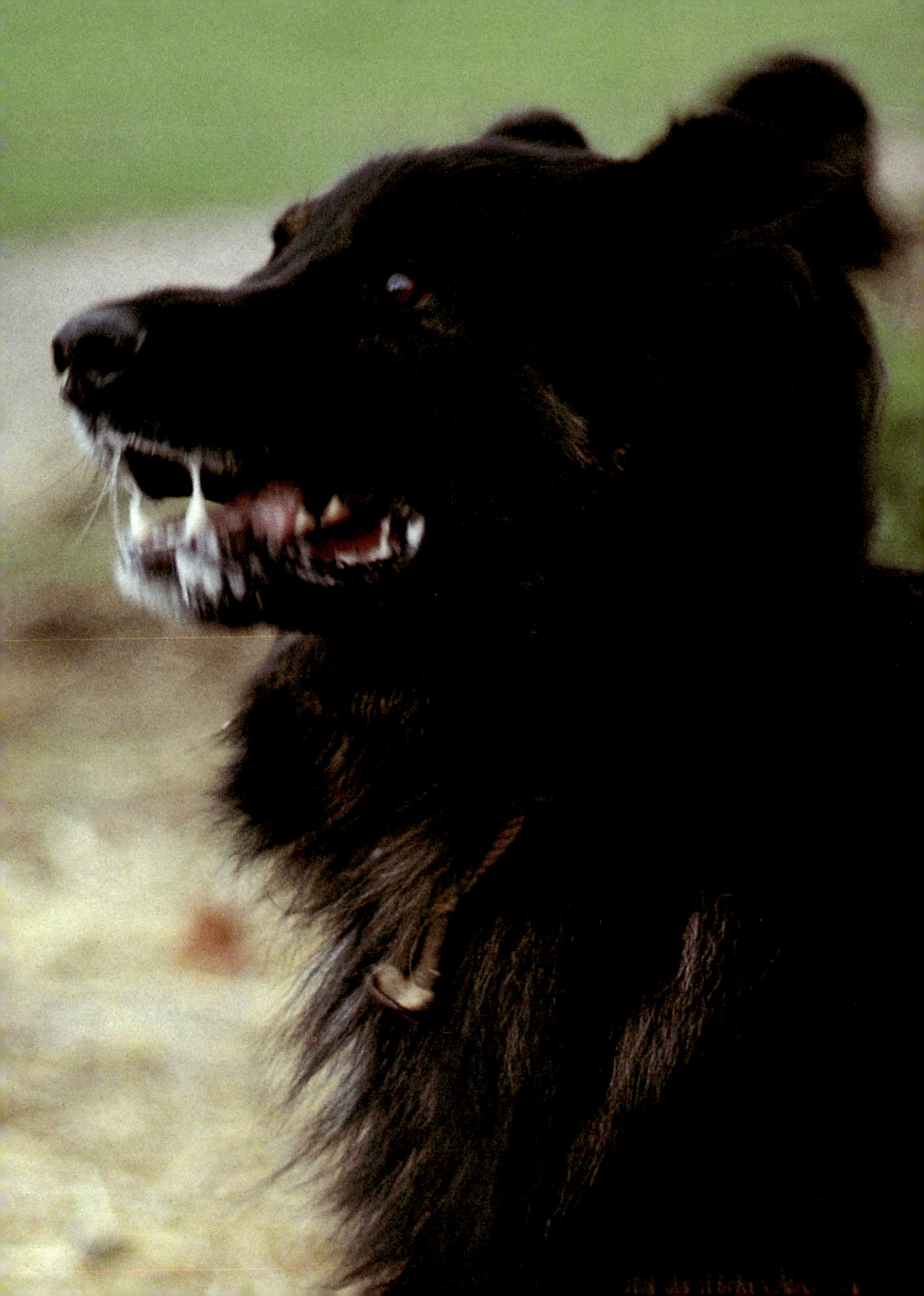

CHAPTER 1
PETS BEHAVING BADLY

Animal behaviour is one of the most interesting aspects of my work – probably because I am so interested in people anyway and because so many owners come to see me about a problem that is rooted in behaviour rather than disease. Sometimes the behaviour is entertaining, sometimes it is curious and sometimes it is downright frightening, but the more you understand why an animal behaves in the way that it does, the easier it is to deal with it and relate to the animal. Very often that means finding out what the animal's natural behaviour would be in the wild; for instance, dogs are domesticated wolves and still behave very much as wolves do.

These days there are specialists who can help you with your pet's behavioural problems, but the most reliable ones will only accept you as a client through your vet. So the first step is to go to the surgery and discuss the problem with your own vet, who might be able to help anyway or, if not, might refer you to an animal behaviourist or even to a basic training class if that is more appropriate.

It is not only the owners who have trouble with the behaviour of their pets. Sometimes we vets have trouble as well!

Rocky

One of the most memorable cases I had early in my career was a German shepherd dog called Rocky. I am not at all surprised about his name; most German shepherds and Rottweilers seem to be called Rocky!

He first came in to see me as a little puppy of 12 weeks, really cute and friendly – and massive. I could see he was going to be a hefty dog. He was owned by a very young couple and I suspect that it was the

Some animal behaviour is frightening, especially for children. An understanding of why our pets behave in the way they do makes their behaviour less alarming and easier to deal with.

man who really wanted a German shepherd. A lot of people who keep German shepherds, especially the men, seem to feel it is a macho kind of dog to have. I am probably being unfair, but it seems that many Rottweilers and German shepherds are owned by people who feel that the breed fits their 'image' but unfortunately they don't always know how to handle them.

About eight months after I had first seen him, Rocky came in again, this time to be castrated. I had talked to his owners about socialisation and training him when he was a puppy and so I was quite curious to see what he was like when he came back for castration. I didn't anticipate what would happen over the next couple of hours.

While the owner was there, Rocky behaved perfectly. I had no reason to suspect that he was bad tempered but I should not have let the owner take the dog into the kennels himself. After he had gone, I went to the kennel to get Rocky out for his anaesthetic. It was a walk-in kennel and as soon as I entered it Rocky pinned me to the wall and growled. I have never been so frightened in my whole life! This really big, shaggy German shepherd went totally wild – and exposed all his teeth in a wide grin. His paws were enormous and when he stood on his hindlegs he was taller than me. It was like being face to face with one of those aliens from the movie. I remember thinking how white his teeth were, because he was growling and pulling his lips back. Still, at least I was able to check his teeth at close quarters! Then somehow I managed to push him out of the way and I stumbled out of the kennels. He was hurling himself at the door as I closed it.

I was really lucky that he did not manage to get me but I was badly shaken, and very frightened. I have not been bitten properly yet (apart from by hamsters), so I am still waiting for the day when it happens. All vets have their own stories about how they were bitten – on the face, on the hands and so on – and I am dreading the day when this happens to me.

The only way we could actually get Rocky out of the kennel was to ask the owner to come back. Unfortunately the owner was out when we rang, but his girlfriend was at home. She came over but she could not control the dog at all. It was obvious that the man was the boss. Once we managed to locate him at work and he came to get Rocky out of the kennel, the dog turned into a little lamb.

It is amazing to see how these dogs become completely different animals once the owner is about. It is easy to understand that, but it is worrying for vets because we are always working with animals that know they are in an unfamiliar situation, and we have to rely on them trusting us. Of course, we have muzzles and, yes, I do muzzle an animal if I have doubts about its reactions; it isn't worth taking risks. It is better for the animal, it is better for my nurse and it is better for me – I have to work with my hands for the rest of my life and I do not want to risk being bitten and damaging my hands. An animal that is frightened or in pain is unpredictable.

So that I could give Rocky his anaesthetic, I had to ask the owner to hold him and the dog was as good as gold. I discussed the aggression with him and he told me that Rocky had big problems with other dogs. He also had a lot of problems with the owner's girlfriend; she, as we had already seen, could not handle the dog at all. He had done nothing about it simply because he didn't know where to start.

It is tricky when you have a large and dangerous dog that is perfectly happy with one person but cannot stand anyone else. I feel strongly that anyone who gets a big dog like a German shepherd or a Rottweiler should go to formal training classes with them. I always emphasise how important it is to be strict with puppies and to make sure that they socialise and also that they are submissive with all members of the family. Otherwise you end up with a perfectly healthy dog that has to be put to sleep at a very young age simply because you cannot cope with its behaviour.

What about re-homing it instead of putting it down? Well, who would want to take on a dog with a difficult temperament? None of the homing charities could take the risk of re-homing an aggressive dog. It is the responsibility of the puppy's owner to make sure that their pet develops into a dog that can mix safely with people and other dogs, and it is usually the fault of the owner, not the dog, when that does not happen.

Types of aggression

You really cannot keep an aggressive dog, especially if it is a big dog and you have small children. Smaller dogs get away with it more than the larger dogs for obvious reasons – it is much more difficult to live with a big aggressive Rottweiler than a little aggressive Yorkshire terrier. The little breeds may do less damage but it does annoy me quite a lot that people do not take their aggression seriously. You end up with snappy little dogs, and that is why some of the small breeds have a bad reputation.

There are different types of aggression. There is the 'dominant aggressive' dog that just looks into your face, looks you in the eye, and he will be absolutely fine as long as you don't do anything to him. Once he has had enough, he will try to get you. This is the very dominant type of animal that has been allowed to be 'top dog' at home and has become used to it.

That kind of aggression can sometimes be dealt with if the owner is the right person and willing to take the risk. Dogs like these are absolutely not suitable for families with small children – it is not worth the risk – but they might be suitable for a single person who is willing to spend time working with the dog and making it realise that it is not meant to be top dog in the human world.

The other type of aggression I see often in the surgery is 'fear aggression'. It is very typical in border collies and also sometimes in springer spaniels and German shepherds. I am careful with some German shepherds because they can become really frightened in the surgery, but at the same time they are very dominant and protective.

With fear aggression, you realise that the dog is worried and it does not really want to hurt you but it does not understand why you are doing what you are doing to it in the surgery. As far as the dog is concerned, it is in hell when seeing a vet and it will do anything to survive. So I sympathise with the dog; it is a pity, but it is just something we have to handle.

The alpha dog

One day I was called out to put another German shepherd to sleep because he was aggressive. He was about four years old. The owners had tried to cope with the situation but could take no more. Basically the dog had taken over the whole house. He had started off by sleeping in the owner's bed, which suited everybody when he was a puppy but then he started to grow up and became more protective about the female in the family. He started to growl at her husband and even

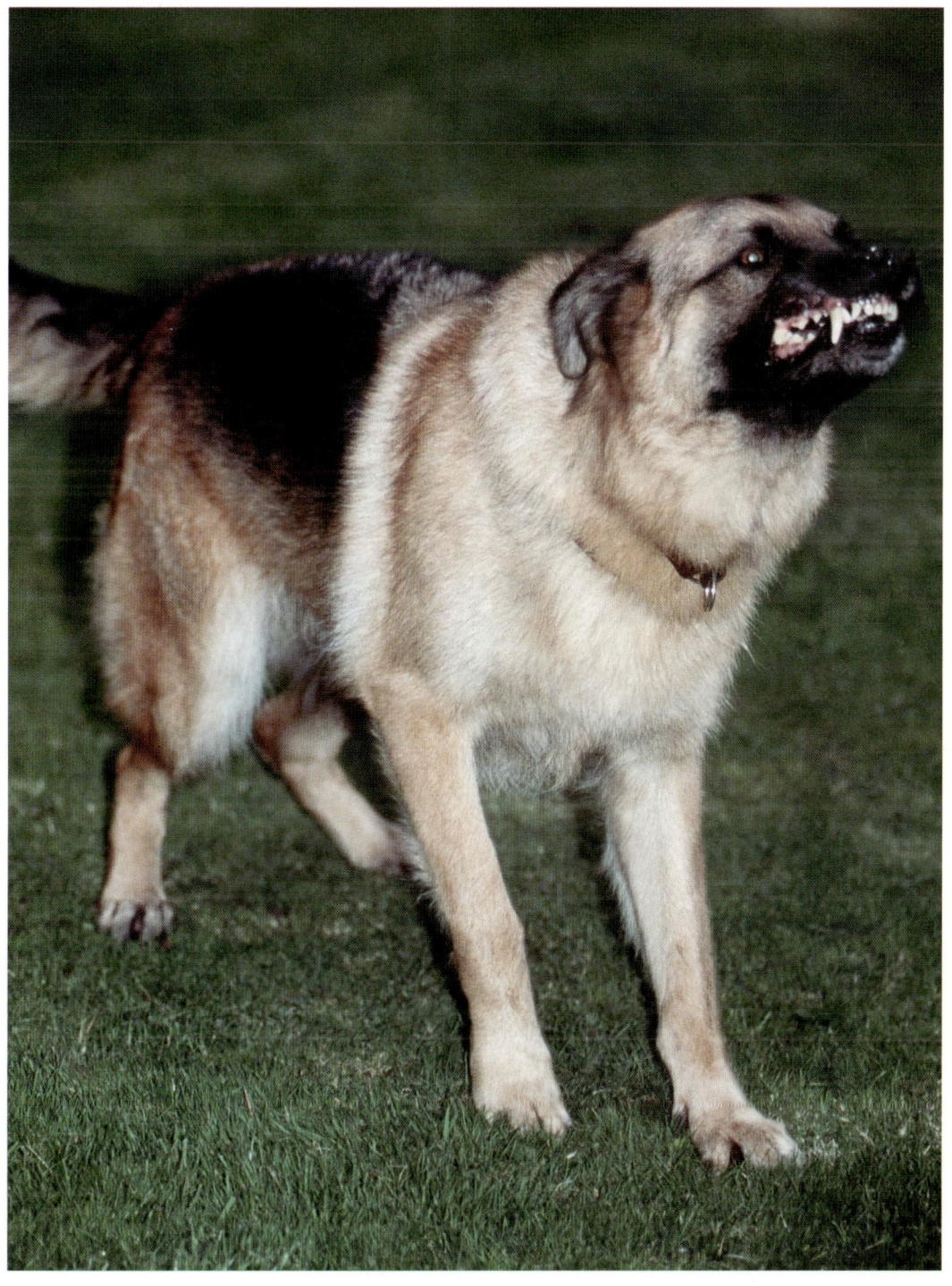

German shepherds are big. Sometimes big dogs are so aggressive they are difficult to control.

stopped him from sleeping in the bed. They were too frightened to remove him from the bed, and so the husband had to sleep on the couch. The next stage was that the dog refused to let either of them come into the kitchen because he would guard it; he would guard different areas, he would guard the sofa, he would guard his food, and he would bite anyone who came too close.

This behaviour is completely natural in the wild for an 'alpha' dog in a pack. Alpha dogs are very dominant; they will give signals to submissive dogs: 'Don't come near this, this is mine,' and so on. But domestic dogs are not living in the wild. Dogs are living with *us*, and it should be on our terms. I always worry when people say they let their dogs sleep on the bed and so on. They might have had a series of dogs for 20 years and they have always been fine, but then one day they have this one dog with a strong dominance streak – and suddenly the husband (or wife!) is sleeping on the sofa.

The bickering bitches

Some time ago I dealt with a case where two bitches lived together and had started fighting each other. The older bitch, a collie cross, had been in this household for about eight years before her owner bought the new puppy, which was a Rottweiler. They were fine at the beginning, until the new puppy reached sexual maturity. When she was about a year old, the fighting started.

The problem was that the younger dog was trying to take over the dominance role from the older one and the older dog was not going to stand for it, so they ended up fighting all the time. It seemed to me that the young puppy had such a dominant temperament that she did not want to back down, which is what would usually happen. Her fighting was quite vicious.

The bitches tended to come in to my surgery at regular intervals with different fight wounds and I had to advise the owners about what they might do to stop the fighting. These situations are quite difficult, especially with bitches. It can be tricky to mix them where there are dominance problems between them and they do not seem to be able to decide who should be dominant and who should be submissive. Usually an age difference will sort that one out, but then sometimes you have 'alpha' dogs with a really strong dominance streak and they will persist in trying it on, trying to take over. In the wild, an old animal will be constantly challenged by young animals and that is just the way it is, because that is best for the pack. Eventually you get a new, fresh, fit and healthy individual taking over.

In this situation, they had to find a new home for the Rottweiler. There was another example of bickering bitches, this time a shih tzu being beaten up by a younger lhasa apso in a household where there were six or seven dogs. The owner was well aware that her animals had the social structure of a pack and was able to talk about it at some length. She certainly knew her dogs and knew that the younger animal would have to go elsewhere if the two bitches could not sort out the situation between themselves.

What should people do when animals fight? The best remedy is to try to predict the situation and avoid or prevent it. If it happens anyway, it happens – it is no one's fault. What you should *not* do is to try to grab hold of the animals. You will get bitten. It is difficult to avoid being bitten if two dogs really go for each other, because they will be so intent on the fight that they let nothing get between them. The best action, if at all possible, is to try to distract them. A bucket of water is often effective; so is a sudden loud noise.

If you walk your dog on a lead and a loose dog approaches you, that can be a potentially bad situation because your dog will feel vulnerable, protective and quite worried that he is on a lead and the other dog is not. You will very often find that dogs that seem to be aggressive towards other dogs when you have them on a lead will be fine if you

Trude's helping hand

What to do about aggressive dogs

- On average, 6000 postmen get bitten by dogs every year, even when they follow Royal Mail guidelines about dealing with difficult dogs.
- Dog owners should be responsible for their dog's behaviour.
- There are different types of aggression in dogs – 'dominant aggression' and 'fear aggression'. If your dog is aggressive then get help as soon as possible. Dog aggression can be sorted out.

TRUDE MOSTUE + **Pets in Practice**

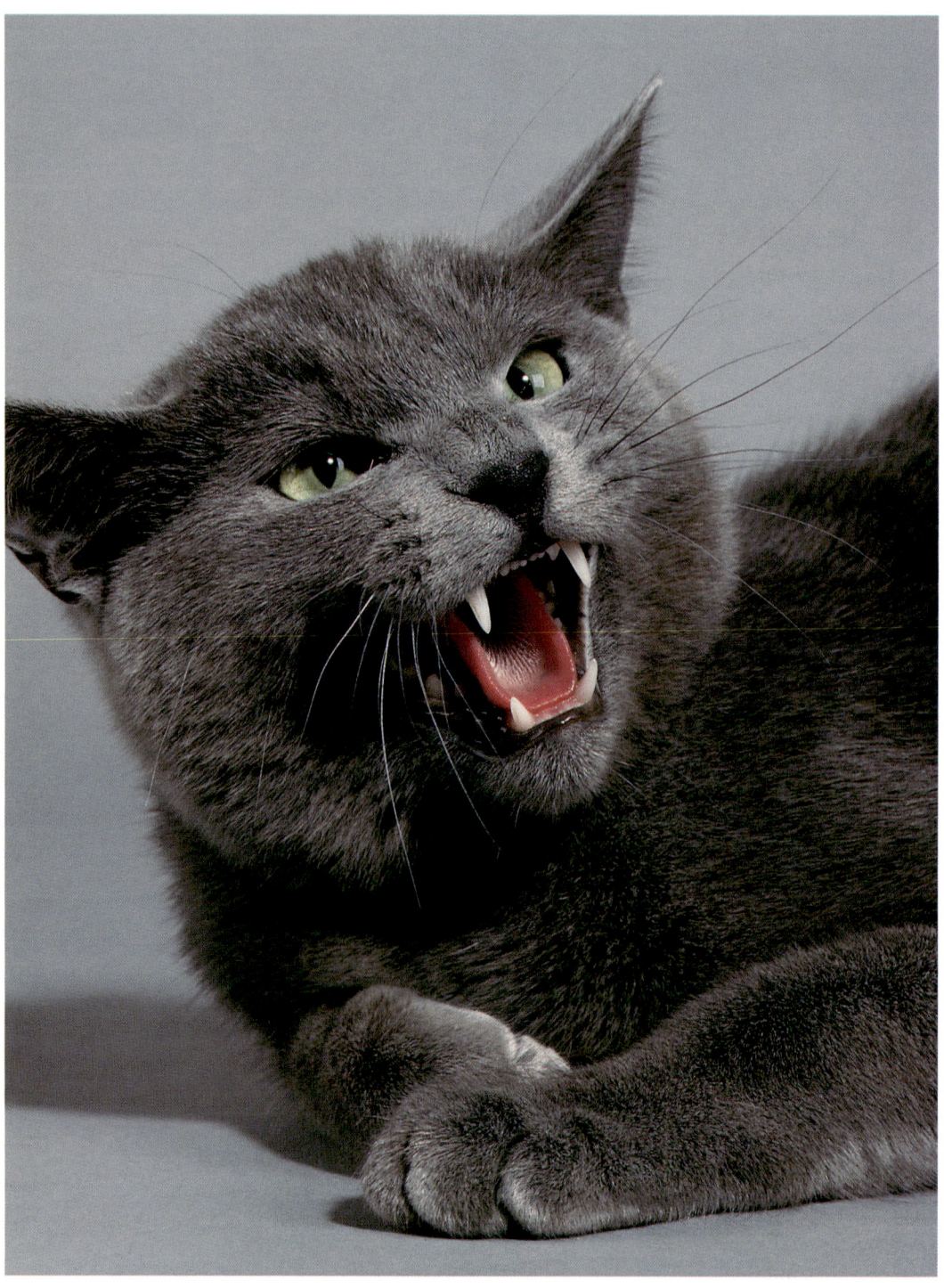

Aggressive cats are quite common. Be very careful with cat bites – they can be nasty and lead to infection.

let them off the lead, so that they can sort out who should be the boss. In that case, usually one dog will become submissive and the other one will act out the dominance behaviour and there will be no fighting.

In general, maybe people do interfere too much and are a little too nervous about what their animals are going to do. Nobody wants to end up in trouble and being blamed for anything, and certainly nobody wants to see their dog being bitten by another in a fight that ends in stitches at the surgery and tears for the owner. But most dogs are really good at sorting out a 'pecking order' between them without actually fighting – unless both of them are dominant by nature, especially if they are bitches.

Plenty of dogs do come in with traumatic injuries from fighting. This is not organised dog fighting, of course, but typically a dog has attacked another one on a walk. The most common injuries are around the neck, because that is where they often try to bite each other. Most of them are puncture wounds and these can be quite serious, because they can induce abscesses – just like cat bites do. Cats have some awful bacteria on their teeth and these can induce very nasty reactions and infections and, in the worst cases, abscesses. Cat-bite abscesses are one of the most common diagnoses we do in the practice in the week.

Sam the border collie

A lot of the behavioural problems we see are due to over-nervousness with new objects and new situations. Some breeds are naturally more nervous and suspicious than others. They need more attention than others, but they are adaptable and you can make them less nervous.

For example, for the weekly column I write for a Scottish newspaper, many of the readers seem to live in rural areas and many of them have problems with border collies. One letter in particular grabbed my attention and it is a good illustration of behavioural problems connected with housetraining and with anxiety in unfamiliar surroundings.

This small family had given a home to a five-year-old border collie called Sam. Sam had originally been on a sheep farm but for various reasons he could no longer work and so he retired to live with this family in a less rural area. The mum in the family complained because Sam did not seem to respond to anything. First of all, he was not housetrained, and she asked why this should be at his age and how she should tackle the problem.

I have come across several cases like this. People do not seem to realise that the life and training of working dogs are totally different from those of pet dogs. Sam had probably lived outside in a kennel all his life; he had probably never been inside a house and so, of course, he had never been housetrained. He would not know the difference between a carpet indoors and the grass outside, and he would certainly not know where *not* to go to the toilet.

Sam also had other problems. He chased the postman; he became very anxious when he was shut indoors; he was frustrated at being limited to regular exercise routines; and he was also frightened every time the phone rang, or when visitors came into the house – he would bark frantically. This was hardly surprising. On the farm he would have had only limited contact with people and he had met only one other dog (the other working collie on the farm). Many working dogs are poorly socialised, especially those that live on isolated farms where they don't see many people. On top of that, if they have never lived in a house they will not be used to the phone or the television, and will be scared by them. So they will bark and be nervous and it will take them some time to get used to these strange things, which is understandable.

Sam's new family also found that he would nip the children's heels when they were running around the house. Yes, of course he would, because he was a sheepdog! As far as he was concerned the children were the flock, and he was herding them in the way he had been trained.

I usually find that it is the dogs that have been very poorly socialised when they were puppies that have a problem with other people and other dogs. I cannot emphasise enough how important it is to socialise your puppy when it is as young as possible – to dogs, to people, to trains and aeroplanes, to crowded streets, to anything. People can be too protective of their pets, not letting them mix, but they should work hard on socialising them when they are young. It will make life so much easier later on.

As for Sam, I explained to the family why he was behaving as he was and my advice to them was to provide him with an outside kennel or something similar – something that was familiar to him from his life on the farm – and then gradually get him used to coming into the house but with the option of going back to his kennel, where he would feel safe.

They wrote to me later to tell me that he was getting on much better, which was really nice to hear.

Yet in many ways I feel that taking on ex-working animals as pets is not always the best solution. You should really know what you are taking on before you make up your mind. I would never recommend a family to take on a dog like this, unless they are well aware of the potential problems. It will take a long time to housetrain the dog, for a start, and in certain cases you never will. It is the same with retired greyhounds: they will not have been housetrained, they need a lot of exercise with a very fit owner, they are probably suffering from old racing injuries and there is the additional problem that racing greyhounds are bred to chase anything fluffy – including your neighbour's kittens!

Living with Lizzy

Separation anxiety is a common behavioural problem in both dogs and cats. They just cannot bear being left on their own and dogs become very destructive. The first time I came across a case like this was actually with my own sister, Lene, in Norway. Lene bought a two-year-old German shepherd called Lizzy. She had a lovely temperament and a very good pedigree, but the owner had forgotten to tell my sister that Lizzy was not used to being on her own during the day. She had grown up with a big family where the wife was always at home.

In Norway it seems to be more common that dogs are left on their own during the day and, as Lene works, Lizzy had to stay at home alone for a little while. My sister had made her a little outside pen and shelter, which is fine for a dog of that size and with a thick coat, but she soon discovered for herself that Lizzy was not at all used to being on her own indoors. She chewed up everything – Lene's sofa, her curtains, her carpets, the door – nothing was sacred.

German shepherds are typical of dogs that are very dependent on having company. It is a disaster for them when people leave them, and they become extremely anxious, worried and frightened. That is when they start to become destructive, in pure frustration.

Lene began to lose her patience after a while. She wanted a dog but she could not afford to replace the sofas and curtains and she could not take Lizzy to work with her; she is an engineer and she could not go to meetings with a dog in tow. So we decided to provide Lizzy with a little sanctuary of her own within the house, where she could stay if she was worried about anything and when Lene went to work.

There is no reason why you should let your dog roam freely around in your house; you can restrict them to one room, as long as they have food and water and a pleasant place to sleep. So Lene restricted her dog to one room and put a big travel cage in there, which Lizzy could go into whenever she wanted. It worked wonderfully. Actually she found out later that she was used to sleeping in a cage.

It was all to do with Lizzy's feeling of insecurity. She was so worried and everything was new – she did not know the house, she did not know the routines, she did not know when Lene would be coming home again. Once she started to get used to Lene and her house, she settled down well. She chose to use the cage herself every time Lene went to work; she felt so much safer in it.

The secret is to think about why the dog is behaving in this destructive way. Usually it is because it is frightened and the key to dealing with the problem is to give the dog a sense of security. A pen of a suitable size might be the solution: it worked for Lizzy and it could be worth trying with your own dog.

There are some drugs on the market that might help in a case of separation anxiety, but I would only use them in difficult cases. It is best to discuss the problem with your veterinary surgeon or animal behaviourist to see whether they think drugs are useful or necessary.

Chloe the Siamese

Separation anxiety is less common in cats, as most of them are more interested in where they live than with whom, but the oriental breeds are slightly different. They are much more likely to be dependent on people and can become neurotic when separated from their owners.

Chloe the Siamese had been living in the same house for about 10 years. Her owner came to see me because, she said, the cat had started spraying all over the house, particularly on her duvet and her expensive jacket. Also Chloe had started to soil under the sofa, on the floor and so on. The owner was becoming desperate and was almost willing to give up; she had been fighting with the problem for several months, trying to put up with it, trying to find out why she was doing it, and she just could not understand why her cat had suddenly started to behave like this.

TRUDE MOSTUE + Pets in Practice

One problem, I discovered, was that a big new estate had just been built not far from where they were living and with that came a lot of new cats. It was not hard to realise that Chloe was responding to these intruders: she was clearly frustrated because they were trying to take over her garden. They were looking for their own territory and it was all very confusing and unsettling for a cat who had lived there all her life.

As we talked it became more and more obvious that Chloe was extremely dependent on her owner and I could see the strength of the bond between them. She was the only cat and had been with her owner since kittenhood. While she was growing up the owner had been at home all the time, because she also had a baby, and so the cat was used to her being at home from the very beginning. But within the past year she had started to go back to work and Chloe had to spend much more time on her own.

Animals, particularly cats, respond to insecurity and show that they are worried by changing their normal behaviour, and the first thing that usually goes wrong is where they urinate and where they defecate. I soon found out that Chloe did not really spray; it was more that she was urinating and defecating everywhere.

It was clear that Chloe's behaviour resulted from her deep anxiety about being on her own during the day. Chloe's problems would take a long time to resolve and a lot of patience. The important thing was to build up her confidence and make her feel more secure.

First of all we tried giving her a little cage so that she could have her own little den inside the flat to make her feel safer if there was a cat outside in the garden. Also the owner started going out into the garden with her

Separation anxiety is most common in oriental cat breeds which are more dependent on people for their happiness than other breeds.

19

before she went to work and when she came home again. This could only be a temporary measure but it did begin to build up Chloe's confidence, so she could start afresh and and feel more secure when she was in the garden with the other cats.

The owner did continue to work, of course – you cannot just put your life on hold because the cat is responding badly to it. We felt that the best and only answer was to try to adapt the cat to her new situation. We discussed getting another cat to keep Chloe company during the day but my worry was that it would make her even more insecure about her territory and would reinforce the soiling behaviour.

It took about three months to build up some improvement. It was a combination of patience from the owner, making sure she made a lot of fuss of Chloe before she went to work and when she came home from work. She provided the cat with her little hiding place and a fresh litter tray; and she cleaned the carpet with a biological cleaner to remove any smell, because the cat would otherwise return to the place that smelled. All these factors combined together worked really well and Chloe is now a much happier and more confident cat.

Barky Sparky

Excessive barking is incredibly common. The first case I dealt with was a fat little black dog. She was really overweight; she was one of those dogs whose head just did not fit with her completely round body – her small head seemed to disappear into a fat neck so that she looked rather like a tortoise. Most overweight animals put a lot of fat on the body and nothing on the legs and nothing on the face, so they look as if they have tiny heads and skinny little legs.

Sparky's owner had not come in to discuss her weight problems, but her barking; she was barking all the time and driving the family crazy. They were really frustrated, because Sparky had been behaving like this for about four years, which meant that it had become a habit that would be quite hard to break. She barked at the postman, she barked when the phone rang, she barked if someone came to visit, she barked at everything. Barking was her main way of responding to everything.

Excessive barking tends to be a way of seeking attention. On a television programme once we were discussing this problem with an elderly couple and their little dog was standing on the table. He kept on barking and barking, and in the end we could not use the piece because nobody could hear anyone over all the barking. Every time he barked, the owners tried to shut him up by giving him a piece of chocolate, so every time he barked he was given a reward.

Rewarding the wrong behaviour is quite a common fault to make. For instance, when I see animals in my surgery, if a dog barks at me and growls at me, lots of owners will give it a little titbit and say, 'Oh poor you, don't worry, don't worry, you'll be fine.' In other words, they are reinforcing the dog's bad behaviour. That is so wrong. People do not realise what they are doing and I have probably done it myself with various animals without realising.

If a dog has a behavioural problem of any kind, you should follow the basic principles of training: reward good behaviour and ignore bad behaviour – but you must be consistent in this. An obedient dog that you can train to sit and roll around and do various tricks can in theory also be trained not to bark. If you can train it to bark, you can train it not to bark. Basic training should start very young anyway and wrong behaviour in young dogs should be dealt with long before it becomes a habit, as it had with Sparky.

> ### Trude's helping hand
> #### *Facts about bad behaviour*
> - The most common behavioural problem in cats is spraying and soiling in the house.
> - The best age for socialising a puppies and kittens is as soon as possible after vaccination.
> - Badly behaved dogs can be cured by training: reward good behaviour, ignore bad behaviour.

Sometimes it is difficult to alter behaviour by telling an animal off. For example, your dog always barks when the postman is coming; you tell it to stop barking and you get really angry. From the dog's point of view, your reaction means it is getting your attention, which is actually a reward for that dog. You might see it as a negative thing, but the dog sees it as a positive thing.

Perhaps what you really need is a device that deters the animal in a gentle way every time it behaves badly. There are various things on the market that seem to be quite effective, working on the principles of rewarding good behaviour and ignoring or gently punishing bad behaviour. For example, there is a collar that squirts some citrus smell in front of a dog's nose every time it barks, which seems to work well: whenever it barks, this squirts in front of its nose, surprises it, and so it stops barking. When it is quiet, you give it a little titbit, so at the same

TRUDE MOSTUE + Pets in Practice

time you are gently punishing bad behaviour and reinforcing good behaviour. Dogs quickly make the association: barking is not nice and being quiet is yummy!

Persistent barking can be quite difficult to deal with; it does take a long time to change the dog's behaviour and needs a lot of patience. I tried to explain to Sparky's family that one of the first things they must do was to stop reinforcing the bad behaviour. They should pay her no attention when she was barking. But I do not think they had the time to do all the little things that were needed. For example, I suggested that one way of punishing her when she was barking was to take her to another room and ignore her, but apparently she barked even more.

She had been barking for so many years that she was not readily susceptible to change and it would take ages to alter the habit.

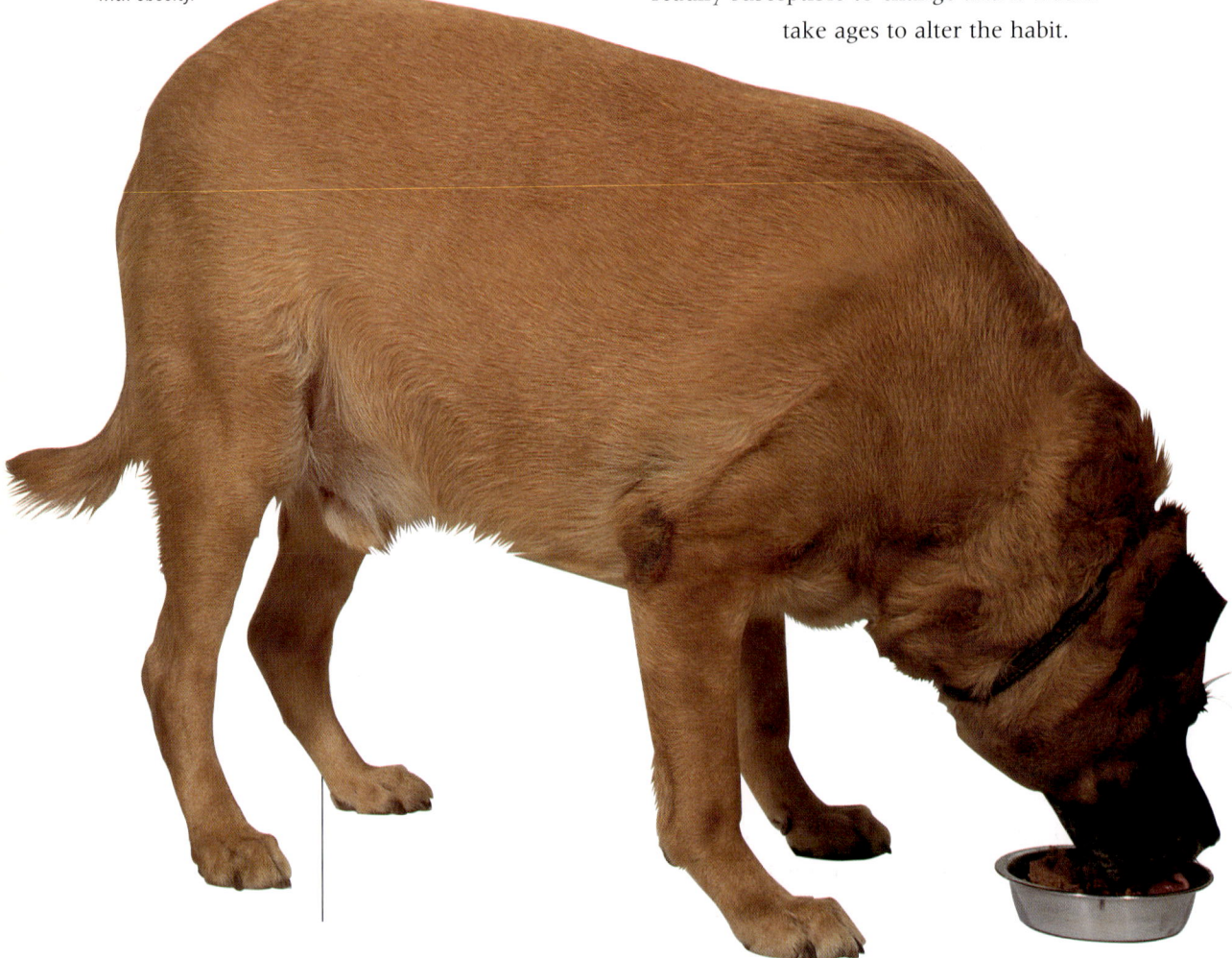

Rewarding dogs with extra food for behaving well is quite common, but can lead to problems with obesity.

Of course, for Sparky, barking was her way of communicating. Like most dogs, she could not see anything wrong with barking. We might find that barking hurts our ears and is in general annoying, but for a dog it is a means of communication. The secret is to find a different way of communicating.

Tigger and the baby

Tigger was a male tabby. He had been a rescue cat and had lived with his present owners for about two years when suddenly there was a new baby in the house. Tigger began to spray – he sprayed on furniture, he sprayed on curtains and he sprayed on his owners' shoes and leather jackets, which did not make him very popular at home. He was brought in to me to find out what could be done.

Soiling the house and spraying on curtains and furniture are the most common behavioural problems I see in cats. Spraying is different from ordinary urinating: with spraying, the cat stands rather than squats and it squirts urine more or less horizontally, usually against an upright surface and quite forcefully, with its tail all atremble. It is normally a way of marking out the cat's territory and leaving messages to other cats to keep away.

Spraying indoors suggests that the cat is a bit mixed up. It is not an easy problem to solve and the secret is to find the cause of the cat's change in behaviour. It is mostly a territorial matter and is often caused by a cat's insecurity over intruders. Usually cats start to spray because they are frustrated about their territory or feel that their territory is threatened – by a new person in the family, an unfamiliar visitor staying in the house, or new cats in the neighbourhood making the resident cat feel insecure about its own territory. A new cat actually in the household is a classic trigger for spraying, and another typical problem is when neighbouring cats come through the catflap and eat the resident cat's own food, making the poor thing very worried and confused. The cat usually lets the intruders get away with it but starts to spray around the door and around the kitchen, just to say, 'This is *my* territory – keep off!'

Tigger's problem was that his 'territory' was being invaded by the new baby, who had started to crawl around on the floor. So Tigger started to spray, even though he had been neutered. Many people think that neutered cats will not spray, but I promise you they will! Neutering might improve the situation but the territorial instinct in neutered cats remains very strong, and so you can expect to see some territorial behaviour in them if they feel challenged.

There are several ways in which you can try to deter a cat from spraying, but above all you need to have patience. First of all, clean the sprayed places thoroughly, but never use ammonium-based products: they simply encourage the cat to spray there again. Use the right type of biological cleaner instead.

That was the first step with Tigger's owners. The next step was to use a clever new commercial product that mimics one of the pheromones secreted by cats. The pheromone relaxes them and seems to assure them that everything is fine, making them feel calmer. I often put this liquid on my hands when I am handling nervous cats and they do seem to respond to it. So I suggested that Tigger's owners should put some of the liquid on the curtains and other places where he was spraying most frequently.

The most important step of all was to try to remove the cause of Tigger's behaviour. Now, obviously that is not very easy to do in the case of a baby! Instead, I suggested that Tigger should be encouraged to make friends with the baby. Perhaps they could start by putting some of the pheromone liquid on the baby's clothes so that Tigger would regard it as something friendly.

Another trick would be to restrict Tigger to a certain part of the house – the kitchen for example – and make sure that the baby didn't go there until Tigger could regain his confidence in his territory. Then gradually the baby could be introduced back into the kitchen and gradually Trigger could be allowed back into the rest of the house.

It is a tedious process, as with all behaviour problems, and it takes a lot of patience and time to sort out. It's always important to remember that the better behaved your pet is, the more you will love it. So it really will be worth it in the end; and you, your baby and your pet will all be happier for it. After all, a loving pet is worth a lot of trouble.

Angry cats and rumbling rabbits

Cats can be even worse than dogs when they are aggressive, although in many ways it is easier to live with an aggressive cat than with an aggressive dog. With a dog you have to interact all the time – you have to put on its lead and take it for a walk, you have to feed it – and dogs in general are very dependent on you. Cats are not: they sleep, they eat as they like, they come and go as they like.

It amazes me how so many people put up with really aggressive cats. I find it quite hilarious, actually! Cats get *such* a good deal. They can get away with being ridiculously grumpy; they can get away with biting or lashing out if you try to touch them; just as long as they purr and sit in your lap once in a while they can get away with it. People say, 'Well, she's all right really because, you know, she does sit on my lap now and then and she does purr. But then the next second she will bite me and she will not let me handle her at all.' Perhaps cats are very clever: they get what they want. And at least cats will give you some warning, and then simply walk away.

Isn't it strange? So many human beings are so desperate to be liked that they are willing to cope with an aggressive animal like that. Some of the cats that come in to my surgery behave really badly and the owners tell me, 'No, no, we can't touch the cat!' (It can be the same with small dogs: it is amazing how much they can get away with.) As long as there are no young children in danger, and as long as you make sure that you can do what you need to do with this animal, then I suppose there is nothing wrong with it, but time after time I am surprised at how many people are willing to put up with really bad-tempered animals and it really is unnecessary.

Some animals are only aggressive when they come and see us – fear aggression. I can understand if owners are prepared to put up with it, but the problem is what *we* have to put up with. We do have our own methods for handling difficult animals, we have muzzles and we have good animal handlers, but badly behaved animals do make our jobs more difficult strangely it's not always the big ones that are the worst. In fact, I am more frightened of hamsters than I am of cats and dogs anyway, so there you go.

I am not saying that every animal that is bad-tempered should be put to sleep but I still think it is extraordinary how many people also feel guilty about it. They should not feel guilty, but what they should do is to train animals when they are young and take the training seriously so that they do not end up with unmanageable pets – particularly with dogs, because they can do so much damage.

There are quite a lot of aggressive rabbits about, too, though their temper usually mellows if they are neutered. I have had several clients coming in with rabbits that bite; who make funny rumbling noises and stamp their feet. This behaviour is typical when rabbits reach sexual maturity. Children who are trying to handle them get kicked and scratched and bitten.

Now a rabbit will not do as much damage as a dog or a cat, but it can lead to problems with the rabbit's own husbandry. Because the animal is difficult to handle, it will increasingly be left in its hutch, which means that it will lead a thoroughly miserable life. What is the point of having a rabbit if it just sits in a hutch and cannot be handled? If you have a big garden where it can run around in peace, that might be a different story, but most people only have a hutch and a little run and that's it.

So when people come in and say that their rabbits are bad-tempered, I definitely advise neutering them if they are not already neutered. It usually helps.

Jumpy gerbils and huffy hamsters

Dogs and cats have been domesticated companions for humans for thousands of years, which means that we should all be used to each other by now, yet they still have a lot of behaviour problems – usually because owners just do not understand the real nature of their pets and often treat them like children instead of animals. Sometimes it is the owners who need to change their behaviour, not the pets. I often wonder if I should treat the owners rather than pets.

With 'exotic' pets – which includes everything from little furry mammals in cages to tortoises, cage birds, reptiles, fish and pet spiders – the relationship with humans is a very false one. Most of them have not been 'domesticated' for anything like as long as cats and dogs, if at all, and also they are more likely to be shut up in a cage or aquarium or vivarium, rather than ranging freely as they would in the wild. Also, they are often kept in ones or twos, whereas perhaps they are of a species that in the wild would be part of a much larger group, or they are kept with other animals when in the wild they would live on their own. On top of all of this stress, many owners do not really understand their basic needs – what the animals should eat, for example, or what temperature they like to live in.

TRUDE MOSTUE **+ Pets in Practice**

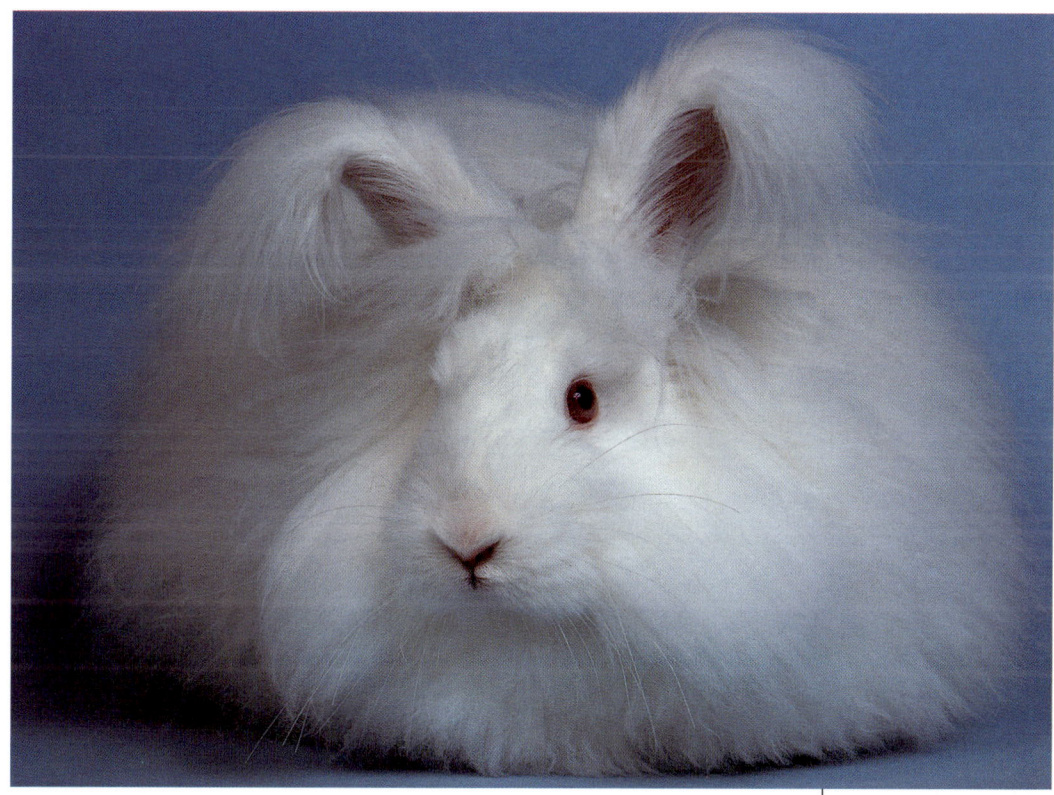

So it is not surprising that quite a number of exotic pets have behavioural problems, though because they are usually small and cannot cause as much harm or damage as, say, a big dog, vets are not often asked about the behaviour problems of a lizard or a hamster or a pet spider.

Quite often those problems will be what is called stereotypical behaviour – repeating the same action again and again and again, like endlessly paddling the wheel – or destructive behaviour of some kind. And very often it is usually through just not knowing, or not understanding, how the animal would behave in the wild and adjusting its environment to take that behaviour into account. The great majority of problems I see with reptiles, for example, can be put down to poor husbandry or poor nutrition.

Let me give you a few examples about the behaviour of small furries and also a few hints that will help your vet when you bring them into the surgery.

Humans have had years of experience in understanding dogs and cats, but more exotic species, such as this Angora rabbit, need extra care and attention as we know less about them as domestic companions.

Gerbils are usually nice little animals, full of curiosity, and they very rarely bite – so I never mind at all when a gerbil is brought in to see me at the surgery. However, you do need to know how to handle them properly. For example, if you try to pick them up by the end of the tail, they will shed the tail skin. If you simply let them sit in your cupped hand they will probably jump off, and rather alarmingly gerbils seems to have no idea about height: they can easily injure themselves by jumping off a table because they think they are only a few inches from the ground. It seems that they have a good head for heights!

Trude's helping hand

Housing for a confined pet

- **Rabbits** are sociable and do not like to be kept on their own. They are quite hardy but need shelter from extreme weather. An outdoor rabbit hutch should be raised off the ground and at least three hops long and tall enough for the rabbit to stand on its hindlegs. There should be as big a run as possible for exercise but make sure the rabbit cannot burrow its way to freedom.

- **Ferrets** are solitary in the wild but in captivity they enjoy company (all of the same sex, or a breeding pair). The hutch can be outside if it is sheltered from the summer sun; it is better to put the hutch in an airy shed. Like rabbits, ferrets need plenty of exercise so a wired run is a good idea as long as it is ferret-proof: they are expert escapologists and can wriggle their way through surprisingly small gaps and holes.

- **Rats**, **mice** and **hamsters** need as large a cage as possible with lots of space for 'furniture' to prevent boredom. Use your ingenuity to create a cage that is more like a wild rodent's burrow, with tunnels and hiding places, but make sure you can clean every part of it at regular intervals. Provide a nest box and appropriate bedding (not the cotton-wool type).

- **Gerbils** often live in a glass 'gerbilarium', placed out of direct sun, half-filled with mixed peat and sawdust so they can create their own burrow system. Give them some nesting material and some cardboard and wood to gnaw.

- **Guinea pigs** are very sociable and should not be kept on their own. Nor should they be kept outside: they cannot tolerate wet weather and are not hardy in Britain. Most guinea pigs are kept in big wooden hutches with two compartments (one solid-fronted for nesting in privacy, the other mesh-fronted for daily living). Like rabbits and ferrets, guinea pigs need plenty of space to exercise and they like to graze in summer, so you could use a rabbit-hutch system with a movable run over the grass. Or you could have a grass run with a piece of drainpipe

Gerbils also tend to panic if you put them on their backs and they often have seizures, which might or might not be a defence mechanism, pretending to a predator that you are dead already so that with luck it will just go away. Sometimes gerbils get into the habit of chewing the bars of their cage in boredom or because their teeth are overgrown, and this can give them mouth sores.

Guinea pigs are usually quite docile, quiet and clean-living but, like most small cage animals, they can easily take fright and then they race around the place. They are easily stressed by extremes of temperature

as a bolt-hole, but put a cover over the run to fend off predators.

- **Chinchillas** can be kept as monogamous pairs or in harems with one male for several females. They need to be kept indoors.

- **Chipmunks** are not house pets: they are best kept in big outdoor aviaries with lots of branches, drainpipes, large stones and so on to play about on.

- **Cage birds** need much bigger cages than most people provide for them. Aviaries are a much better idea if you have the space and if you clean them out regularly. Whether cage or aviary, provide perches of different diameters as well as different heights. If you have a parrot, it still needs a cage even if it has the freedom of a room – the cage is a place it can call its own and where it can feel safe. Parrots, budgies, cockatiels and others in the psittacine group are full of natural curiosity and intelligence, so they do need to keep themselves occupied. They like to be where the action is, so have them

in a room where there is plenty going on. Also remember that most birds are highly nervous of predators, which is why in the wild they like to perch safely out of reach. So the cage is best placed quite high in the room, at or above your own eye-level. It should be protected from draughts and too much direct sunlight, but in a room that is well ventilated.

- **Reptiles** are usually kept alone: they are not social animals. It is very important that you find out precisely what their needs are, especially the temperature and humidity range that best suits the species. Reptiles are kept in temperature-controlled and light-controlled vivariums. Depending on the species, some of them need enough height to climb around in, others need plenty of floor space, and some need bathing water and basking places. All of them like somewhere to hide from prying eyes now and then.

TRUDE MOSTUE + Pets in Practice

I prefer it if small animals are brought in to see me in something like a shoe box – they are usually easier to handle that way. If the animal needs to stay overnight vets always have a number of cages like these for the 'visitor' to stay in.

in their environment, so you need to make sure that it is not too warm or too cold. I would rather people did not bring their guinea pigs in a cage to see me: it is much easier for me to handle them if they are in something like a shoe box.

As for hamsters – well, let us just say that vets have a healthy respect for them! I never quite understand why hamsters are given to children as pets: for a start, they can catch colds from children and also they are nocturnal animals, so all they do during the day is sleep. What is more, they like to live on their own – they are just not very sociable and you can almost guarantee that if there is more than one hamster there will be a fight. They are particularly grumpy if they have just been woken up, and their bite can be really quite vicious and painful, as many a vet knows from experience. Hence the respect!

Hamsters have this neat little trick of fooling you into thinking they are dead. In warm weather they can suddenly go all stiff and just lie there, but if you touch them they usually start trembling and rolling their heads around, then are back to normal within five minutes. On the other hand, in cold weather they might go into hibernation mode and again seem to be dead as their breathing is so slow and shallow that you think they are not breathing at all. If you think your hamster is dead because it is not moving, do not bury it! Either disturb it if the weather is warm, or warm it up carefully on a heated pad for up to an hour if it is cold. If it still seems to be dead after that, it probably is.

Another hamster trick that often alarms owners is that a mother will sometimes hide her babies in her cheek pouches if she thinks they are in danger. Usually she keeps them safe there, but sometimes she really does eat them (charming!)

One of my real concerns with hamsters is those exercise wheels. You would never see a hamster endlessly running like that in the wild for no purpose and it can be dangerously stereotypical behaviour.

Rats n' Mice n' all things nice

I prefer rats and mice to hamsters, though pet mice will also bite if they are in strange surroundings like a veterinary surgery. Again, it is easier for the vet if you bring your mouse in a small container rather than a cage.

Rats very rarely bite unless they are being caused pain or are very frightened. They like to be active and it is quite important to make them and hamsters work a little for their food. It is so boring for them just to be given a big bowl of food. It is much better to hide it in small parcels around the cage (or around the room, if you dare) so that they can search for the parcels and then move the food to wherever they want it. That way, they feel more like a real animal doing something with a purpose.

Most chinchillas are friendly little things, though sometimes rather shy and they do frighten easily. Usually they are easy to handle (they very rarely bite you) and can be picked up gently round the shoulders, in which case you won't cause 'fur slip' (the fur virtually comes away on your fingers). One sign of stress in chinchillas is chewing fur – their own or their mate's. This is usually because they are bored, or their diet is not right, or they feel dirty – all things that the owner could easily make better.

Chipmunks are very different in character to those dear little chinchillas. Chipmunks are very active; they live life at the double, moving very fast, and are experts at climbing out of reach. They need plenty of space, plenty to explore, and plenty to amuse themselves with. In the wild they live on their own and get defensive about their burrow, which means some of them can be quite aggressive. They easily become stressed and none of them seem to like being handled, especially by a vet; their bite can be quite hard! An unexpected problem with chipmunks kept as pets is that television can cause them huge stress. No, it is not the quality of the programmes, but something to do with the frequency of certain sound waves.

Toby the bald parrot

In my first year as a practising vet, I met an African grey parrot called Toby. He used to be handsome but now he did not look very good. All his feathers were gone and the owner said that he would sit there all day literally pulling out his feathers with his beak. When I started to talk to Toby's owner I discovered that his wife, who apparently looked after Toby, had gone into hospital two or three weeks before and it seemed to coincide with the onset of Toby's behaviour.

Poor old Toby was used to being with Mr Brown's wife all day while Mr Brown was at work. Now he was left on his own the whole day and his only company was in the evenings with Mr Brown, who did not feel that the parrot was interested in him anyway, and so he did not give it a lot of attention.

Feather-plucking is quite common in birds in captivity. Usually it is a behavioural problem caused by boredom or frustration, especially in parrots. Many people do not realise that parrots are extremely intelligent birds; they need plenty of mental stimulation, plenty of exercise and plenty of space. In fact parrots, and even cockatiels, should be treated more like a dog than a cage bird, and given as much time and attention as you would give a dog.

The feather-pulling problem can also be caused by viruses or parasites and it is important to exclude those causes before you conclude that it is all in the mind. In this case I took a blood sample and plucked a feather (one of the few he had left!) to check for viruses, mites and other parasites. The results were all negative and we were left with the possibility of a behavioural problem caused by Mrs Brown's absence in hospital.

I discussed the possibilities for a long time with Mr Brown. For instance, he could give Toby a bigger cage, get him out more often, make his environment more stimulating, hide his food around the house so he had to look for it, give him a much more varied diet, and interact with him more. People tend to make life too easy for their parrots and they give them too uniform a diet as well. In the wild, of course, Toby would be flying around searching for food and finding a wide variety. It is very important to find out what the natural behaviour of any species of pet would be in the wild, so that you can understand how best to keep them. For example, African Grey parrots are flock birds and so it is no wonder that they go crazy on their own.

To break the cycle of feather-plucking I put a small plastic Elizabethan collar on Toby and he accepted that quite well; there was a little squeaking and clawing and scratching and trying to eat me but we did manage to do it in the end.

Toby eventually recovered and when Mrs Brown came home from hospital I could see a marked improvement in his behaviour. He is very well now. He still feather-plucks but much less than before. It will take a bit more time to break him of the habit. His attachment to Mrs Brown is quite typical: parrots usually do choose one person they really like and are often aggressive to everybody else. I just hope Mrs Brown never did what some people do in those circumstances, which is to pass food from mouth to beak or even kiss the parrot. Parrots often have psittacosis, a chlamydia infection that can be passed to people long before the bird itself shows any symptoms of the disease. When they do produce symptoms, parrots, cockatiels and budgies often die within a few days. If humans catch the disease, they might just have mild 'flu-like symptoms but in elderly people it can be much more serious and indeed, in some cases, fatal. The organism can also infect dogs, cats and other animals that live in the same house.

Feather problems in cage birds are more usually caused by stress or boredom or overcrowding, rather than parasites or disease, but extra care needs to be taken where the birds are in groups as sometimes a virus might be involved. Of course, it is normal for birds to moult their feathers: usually they will lose some of them at least once a year and this is controlled by hormone levels. But if they just keep on and on moulting, then the hormones are out of balance and you probably need to make their environment a bit cooler and boost their intake of minerals and certain vitamins.

Most of the cage birds I see come in for nothing more serious than claw-clipping. Incidentally, someone has named their budgie after me, but that is another story ...

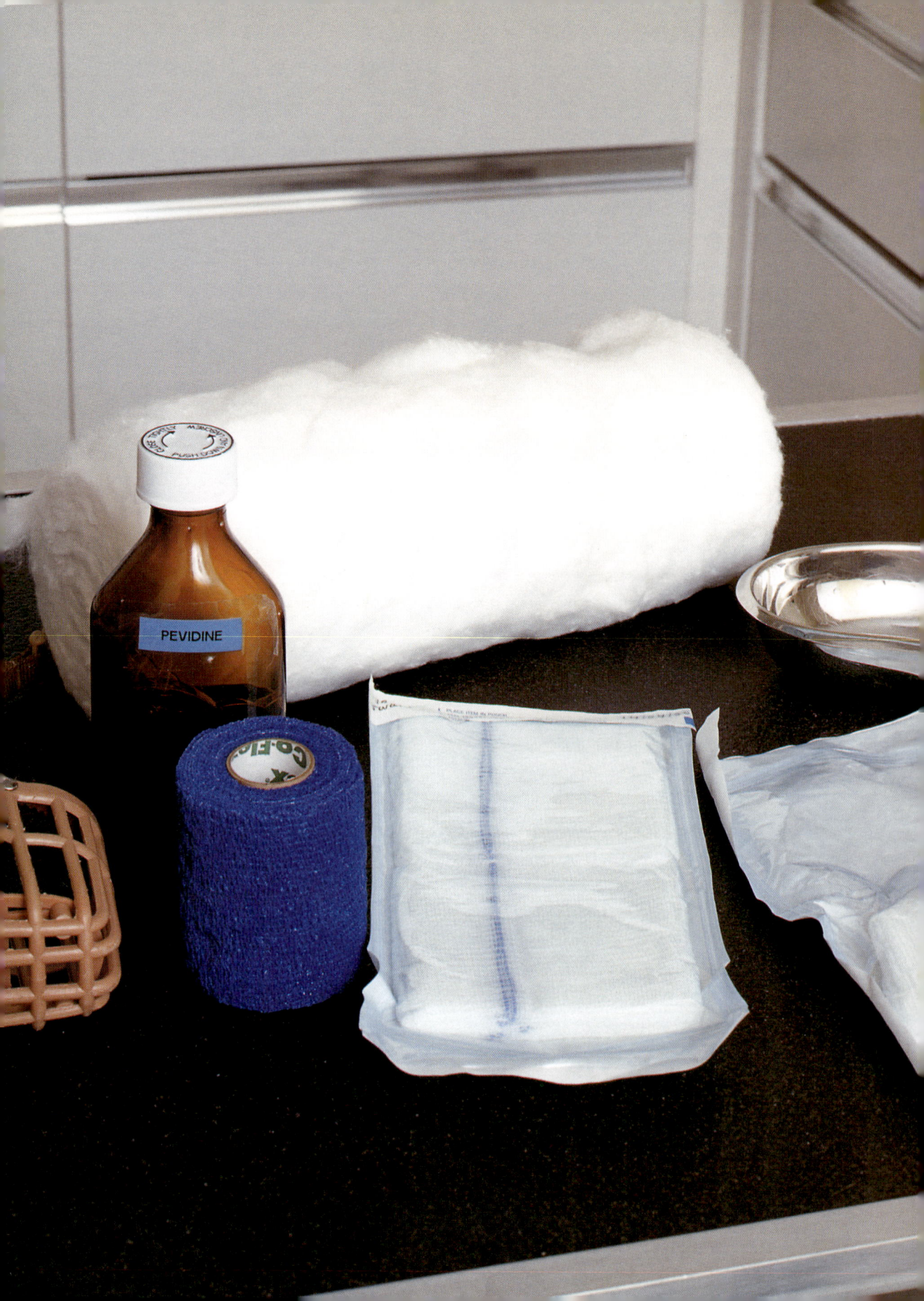

CHAPTER 2
EMERGENCIES

When you work in a veterinary surgery you always have to expect the unexpected (all veterinary surgeries have to offer 24-hour emergency opening, by law). Every now and then someone comes rushing into the surgery in a big panic because something dramatic has happened to their animal – or at least they think it is dramatic and very often it is. Sometimes it goes the other way: a pet is brought in because it does not seem to be quite its usual self, it is a bit off colour – and the next thing you know it is fighting for its life. Some pets, especially the smaller ones and definitely birds, do not give much warning when they are really ill; and with others it seems that the stress of being in alien surroundings in the surgery is almost enough to kill them.

My heart does always start to race a bit when I know it is an emergency, but vets and nurses have been trained to deal with all emergency problems and we all know that there are certain procedures we must follow. The first thing to do is keep calm, draw breath and think very clearly so that you can identify which of the animal's symptoms needs the most urgent treatment. Sometimes it is not the most obviously frightening ones, and sometimes what looks really frightening is not actually an emergency at all. And sometimes what you have to do is calm the owner down as well, whose near-hysteria might be putting even greater stress on the animal (and the vet!)

The most common emergencies I see are from road traffic accidents or fight bites and from poisoning. Many of the other emergencies are avoidable but then, accidents will always happen when you least expect them, however careful you might be.

Vets have to expect the unexpected, and their surgeries are always well equipped to deal with emergencies.

Lucky by name

It was June in my first year in practice at Staple Hill, and it was one of those wonderful, rare weeks when it is really hot. So when an owner brought in her dog Lucky after finding her just lying in the garden, panting, when she came home from work, my first thought was heatstroke.

It happens every summer and particularily if it is hot. They have left the dog in the car while they do their shopping or while they are at some outdoor event, with just a tiny crack of window open (they don't want the car stolen, after all). When they parked the car, it was in the shade of a tree, but they forgot that the sun and the shade would move. Luckily a passer-by noticed that the dog was in a state of collapse from heatstroke, and summoned help from the police and the RSPCA, so the dog was saved. Heatstroke can so easily be fatal.

It is not just dogs in cars. Ferrets are particularly prone to heatstroke: they are not good at losing body heat, they do not sweat, nor do they pant very effectively. Most ferret owners are aware of the problem and realise that they must act very quickly to cool the ferret down by soaking its body in cold water and fanning it at the same time, while heading for the vet at the double. Rabbits can suffer badly at temperatures higher than about 26 or 27°C, and it is essential to ensure that outdoor hutches are not left in full sun. Indoors, birds in cages and fish in tanks can have severe problems with overheating when they find themselves with the sun streaming through the window, and with nowhere to escape from its beams. Dogs only loose heat through panting. Cats have sweat glands on paws and pant when extremely hot.

Anyway, to return to Lucky: she was a brown-and-white collie cross and rather overweight. We took her in and I soon found out that she was fitting. She had an incredibly high temperature, which worried me a great deal, and very soon she started to pass some green diarrhoea. The combination of green faeces and fitting is highly indicative of poisoning from slug bait, if an animal eats enough of the stuff.

Apparently the owner used to leave Lucky in the garden while she went to work. It was an enclosed garden, and she could not understand how Lucky had managed to find the slug bait.

All you can really do in such a situation is to give supportive therapy and try to wash out as much of the poison as possible. One problem was that we had no idea how long it had been since Lucky had eaten the poison, so we tried to wash out her stomach and gave her certain products to make it pass through quicker. We put her on a drip, tried to cool her down and gave her a long-acting anaesthetic to get her out of the fit. It was touch and go – she was so hot and with a temperature that her brain was almost cooking. I was really worried about brain damage, if she survived.

When I left that evening Lucky was lying there, and looking very unhappy and very poorly. The next morning I went to check on her, fearing the worst. To my amazement, she was jumping up and down in her cage and absolutely fine! None of us could believe it. Somehow she had managed to pull through: she had slept through the anaesthetic, she had stopped fitting and her temperature was back to normal. Her name certainly suited her – she was definitely very lucky, against all the odds.

It is so important to make sure that any poisons are inaccessible to pets, including some everyday substances that you might not appreciate are poisonous. Dogs in particular are great scavengers, eating things just to see what they are like, and they are even more notorious for drinking things. Never leave liquids in open containers where dogs can get their noses in, because they will try to drink the contents and the consequences could well be fatal. Garden sheds and garages are full of dangerous substances; for example, anti-freeze for the car tastes sweet and cats sometimes take a fancy to it, with disastrous results.

The only species I can think of that has 'nutritional wisdom' is rats. They have the sense to take just a little taste of something new, and if they feel a bit ill they will never eat that substance again. Dogs, on the other hand, never learn – they'll eat just about anything!

Fits

It is very frightening when an animal has a fit for the first time. Apart from situations such as poisoning, fits (also called convulsions or seizures) usually suggest an underlying disease of some kind unless it is primary epilepsy (epilepsy can be caused by underlying disease like a brain tumor or an animal can have primary epilepsy the cause of which is unknown. The latter can be controlled with tablets. But the former is progressive and can be terminal, depending on the cause.

In dogs they tend to happen after the animal has been asleep; it might wake up suddenly and seem to be anxious, then it collapses, falling over and probably 'paddling' with its feet. If it loses consciousness for more than about 20 seconds, you have an emergency and should contact your vet immediately. Continuous fitting could be *status epilepticus*, a sort of short-circuiting in the brain, and the problem is that there is so much activity in the brain that it reaches a very high temperature. The vet will sedate or anaesthetise the animal to calm the brain and bring it out of the fit.

All you can do at home when an animal is fitting is to keep calm, call your surgery immediately and in the meantime move away any obstacles such as furniture so that the animal does not injure itself when it jerks about during the fit. Make sure that there is no sudden noise. Keep the room dimly lit and do not handle or restrain the animal. Do not drive your pet to the surgery while it is actually fitting; wait until the seizure has finished, because to handle an animal during a fit can be disastrous. Wait until it responds to its name or it tries to get to its feet (if this takes longer than 20 seconds, go to the vets straight away).

Trude's helping hand

What to do if your pet has a fit

- Be careful – the animal's temperament may well become unreliable and you might need to protect yourself.

- If the animal is in a dangerous place (e.g. beside a pond or at the top of a staircase) you need to move it to where it cannot come to harm. To do so and to protect yourself at the same time from an unexpected reaction, throw a blanket over the animal before carefully lifting it away from the danger, or gently push it away with your feet.

- With an animal, you do *not* need to wedge its mouth open with a piece of wood between its teeth to stop it biting its tongue.

- If there are other animals, especially dogs, keep them away until the fit is over: they have been known to attack animals having fits.

- Most fits are not emergencies, but status epilepticus (epilepsy) is and you need veterinary help quickly. If the animal continues to have one fit after another over a period of time, you should be worried.

- One of the major problems with epilepsy is that people stop the treatment. Never stop the medication given to you by the vet for your pet's epilepsy, even if it seems to be better. Almost invariably this will result in worse and more fits.

Terry takes the tablets

A big ginger tom called Terry was brought into my surgery looking very ill. He was only two years old and had been in to see me a couple of days before with quite a poorly leg. He had jumped down from a tree and twisted his leg; he had a swollen muscle and swollen tendons but no fractures showed on the X-ray. So I packed him up and sent him home. He seemed to be content with that.

He looked really fed up when he came back to see me the second time after days later and I was wondering what on earth was happening. He was vomiting and very lethargic but, more scarily, he looked as though he was not really with it. I examined him and the leg did not seem to be causing him a lot of pain, in fact it seemed to be on the mend. I checked his gums, which were quite pale, but I could not work out what was going on.

All the while I was talking to the owner, who happened to say to me, 'Well, it all started after I gave him that paracetamol tablet for his leg.' And I thought, oh no! Paracetamol is poisonous to cats; their livers cannot break it down and so they get really high levels of paracetamol circulating in the blood, causing toxic effects and liver damage. They can actually die from it. I had to act fast...

This is not the case in dogs, which is no doubt why people go wrong. They assume that because you can give paracetamol to dogs, you can give it to cats as well. I knew that Terry's owners only meant to give him some pain relief; they wanted to save money on buying painkillers from us for the cat, and as they had been given paracetamol tablets for the dog a week before they thought that it would not do the cat any harm. They said to me, 'Well, we knew it was either aspirin or paracetamol you can give to cats, but we thought it was aspirin we could not give.' So they had opted for the paracetamol. It was a dangerous mistake. It is essential to remember which is which. If you're not sure then ask your vet before you give your pet any drugs at all.

All I could do was to put Terry on a drip, give supportive therapy and just hope that he would pull through it. He was lucky – he did recover without any problem; but I have seen cats die from paracetamol poisoning.

The most important lesson to learn from Terry's case is the need to be careful with any type of painkiller, especially anti-inflammatories that we use in human medicine. For example, you must not give ibuprofen to dogs or cats. It is safest to have a straight policy of not giving any human painkillers – aspirin, paracetamol or anything else – to animals unless the vet supplies them for a particular animal. It will save you from making a potentially deadly mistake. People often assume that cats and dogs are exactly like humans, which is a very dangerous assumption. Physiologically, the different species are not exactly like us. If you feel you must use a painkiller you happen to have at home, call the vet first to check that it is safe to use and what the dosage should be.

Emergency action if your pet has been poisoned

First, find out exactly what the poison is. Bring the label or the bottle – anything that can tell us quickly what the animal has eaten. Then get to the vet quickly. Whatever the problem, a vet will be able to deal with it quickly and efficiently and will know the appropriate antidote as well as the most effective emergency treatment.

Even if you do know the substance, there is very little you can do at home and some of the usual actions can in fact make matters worse. For example, if a caustic substance has been ingested, you should *not* try to make the animal sick – its throat and mouth will already be badly inflamed and will be made more so if the caustic stuff passes over them again in vomit. In any case, never try to induce vomiting in an animal that is having convulsions; wait until it has recovered.

If you are advised that it is appropriate to make an animal sick, you can give it an emetic. At home, you could use salt and water (about two tablespoonsful of salt in a cup of water), washing soda or Epsom salts. In some cases you need a demulcent to soothe inflamed membranes (at home these might be milk, raw eggs, olive oil or liquid paraffin) and in some cases strong black tea or boiled coffee will help.

Birds and poisoning

Everybody has heard of the old miners' tradition of taking a caged canary down the mineshaft to give warning of unbreathable air down there. Birds are much more sensitive to air pollution than we are, and in fact there are some quite surprising fumes in the home that can poison pet cage birds. Carbon monoxide from vehicle exhaust pipes or badly maintained heating boilers are obvious exaples, but there are also two hidden kitchen hazards: fumes given off by burning fat and fumes given off by overheated non-stick saucepans and frying pans. The fumes from fresh emulsion paint and products used to thin or strip paint do birds no good at all. They are also vulnerable to lead poisoning when they peck at old paintwork in the house, or at the 'leaded lights' you find in cottage windows.

If a bird swallows something poisonous, this is definitely a case for the vet, who will remove poison from the bird's crop or stomach by sucking or washing it out. There are various home antidotes for different poisons but the list is a long one. Very strong cold tea can be useful.

Trude's helping hand

Most common poisons

- Anticoagulant rodenticides (warfarin) are the most common cause of poisoning, especially in dogs. They cause haemorrhage and the clinical signs include swellings under the skin full of clotted blood, pallor, bleeding from the nose, dark tarry faeces, pinpoint haemorrhage in membranes and sometimes fits.

- Vitamin D3 rodenticide is a new rodent killer that causes increased calcium 12–36 hours after ingestion (anticoagulant in 1–3 days), depression, anorexia, vomiting, excessive thirst and a lot more urine than usual.

- Organophosphates, used in pesticides (especially on farms), cause diarrhoea, an increase in urine production, narrowing of the pupils and slow pulse rate.

- Paraquat/diquat herbicides cause irritated mucosae, a staggering gait and breathing difficulties several days after ingestion.

- Metaldehyde slug bait can cause salivation, tremors and, later, seizures.

- NSAIDs (non-steroidal anti-inflammatory drugs) can cause kidney and gastrointestinal and liver problems. Cats are more sensitive to them than dogs.

- Antifreeze (ethylene glycol) tastes sweet and cats seem to be attracted to it. Signs of trouble start about an hour after ingestion and range from depression to staggering, coma and perhaps vomiting and convulsions.

- Household products:
  – Chewed matches: blue gums and tongue and breakdown of red blood cells.
  – Bleach (an inhalation hazard): pain and inflammation of the mouth, throat, lungs and stomach.
  – Perfumes: damages to the liver, kidney and central nervous system.
  – Anti-dandruff shampoos: retinal detachment and other eye problems.

- Lead poisoning, including from lead paint residue, dust from sanding down old paint, ingestion of fishing weights or shotgun pellets (and even curtain weights) or old golf balls or linoleum: can affect gastrointestinal tract and central nervous system; chronic diarrhoea, acute abdominal pain, anorexia.

Trude's helping hand

Emergency treatment at home for poisoning

The aim in dealing with any poison, be it gas and fumes, something swallowed or something injected (venom from a sting), is to reduce the body's absorption of the poison as quickly as possible. Here are some of the actions you can take while somebody else is phoning the surgery.

- **Gases:**
  - Immediately remove the animal from the source of the gas or fumes and into the fresh air. Then check that its air passages are free.
  - If the animal is unconscious or in a state of collapse get veterinary help immediately. In the meantime, if you know how to give resuscitation, do so, but do *not* use mouth-to-mouth techniques as you will probably inhale the poisonous fumes yourself.

- **Ingested poisons:**
  - Acids: Do *not* induce vomiting. Call the vet and in the meantime neutralise the acid with an alkaline demulcent (e.g. bicarbonate of soda in milk) or, if there is nothing else, plenty of water to dilute the acid. Never try to force liquid down the throat of any unconscious animal.
  - Alkalis (e.g. ammonia, caustic soda): Neutralise with a very diluted acid (e.g. weak vinegar).
  - Arsenic: Get to the vet *immediately*. If you cannot, give a strong solution of salt and water to induce vomiting.
  - Baits: For alphachloralose (in baits for woodpigeon and mice) an emetic must be used within half an hour of ingestion and the animal must be kept warm. For metaldehyde (in slug baits) only the vet can help; in the meantime keep the animal quiet and in the dark – it is vital that there are no sudden noises, as the animal will be fitting.
  - Barbiturates: Keep the animal warm, give emetics and strong coffee if it is not unconscious. It might need artificial respiration.
  - Lead: Give plenty of Epsom salts, milk, egg whites or strong tea (but not for birds).
  - Pesticides, herbicides: Get veterinary help immediately. Meanwhile, keep the animal still to reduce circulation of the poison, and keep it warm. Do not induce vomiting. If you know the source of the poison, take the container's label to the vet for details of the contents.
  - Phenols (creosote, pitch, carbolic acid, coal tar antiseptics etc.): These are usually ingested because an animal has the substance on its skin and has tried to lick it off. Swallowing these corrosive substances leads to shock, convulsions and death. Give milk or raw egg white by mouth while contacting the vet.
  - Phosphorus (rat poison, chewed matches): If there is vomit, it will be green and will glow in the dark. Act immediately – death is rapid. The animal will be lethargic but intensely thirsty, with acute abdominal pain and diarrhoea. Give an emetic but do *not* use any oils, fats, egg whites or milk. The best emetic is copper sulphate (bluestone) given every 15 minutes.
  - Strychnine: Violent and frightening symptoms (convulsion, arching backwards). This is extremely urgent – contact the vet immediately. Meanwhile keep the animal in an absolutely quiet environment (the slightest noise or stimulus could be fatal).

Simba the jaywalker

I first met a black-and-white short-haired tom called Simba quite late on a Tuesday night. It was about seven o'clock and I was really tired when I heard over the caller that a road traffic accident victim was coming in. Usually with road traffic accidents you know straight away that you will need to stabilise the animal and begin anti-shock treatment, so I started to prepare an intravenous drip and different kinds of medication.

Simba was brought in by the two Jackson brothers, who were carrying him in a cardboard box. They both had wide smiles with very few teeth. He was only about eight months old but the poor thing looked like a 15-year-old cat. He was just lying in the box as if he were asleep.

It took me a while to establish who the two brothers were and their relationship with Simba. It turned out that he belonged to their mother, who had found the cat just lying in his basket in the morning. He didn't want food and he didn't want to move, and that is why they brought him into the surgery. Nobody had any idea what might have happened to him.

I checked him quickly before I took him into the hospital. I noticed immediately that his breathing was quite fast and strained, and that his head was really swollen and his nose looked as if it had been punched. This is quite common with a road traffic accident – vehicles usually hit them from the side and on the head. I checked his claws and they were all frayed, really broken up; they looked as if they had scraped along the road surface, which is something else we often see with road traffic accidents.

Apart from that I could not discover any broken bones, but broken bones at this stage were not anything I would worry about. Fractures, unless they are bleeding a lot, do not concern us in such an emergency. Much more important are any internal injuries, in the chest and the abdomen. I checked the mucous membrane colours in his mouth and his gums and they were quite nice and pink, so I assumed he was not actually bleeding into his abdomen. As he was breathing quite fast and struggling to breathe properly, I assessed his breathing as being the main emergency problem.

Having explained the procedures to the two brothers, I took Simba into the surgery and put him on a drip. I left the drip running overnight and when I came back in the morning he was still struggling to breathe.

So I gave him a sedative, took an X-ray of his chest and took some blood from him. The X-ray showed that he had pneumothorax, which means air pockets in the chest.

Imagine it like this: the lungs are two sets of sacs. Usually there is negative pressure inside the chest and if there is an injury that causes air to leak into the chest, air pockets will form and compress the lungs inside the chest.

As Simba's condition was not really bad and it was only on one side, I decided to leave him in the cage for a couple of days and see if he improved. The blood samples came back and they showed that he'd had bleeding from his liver, but he was recovering.

All the evidence pointed to a car accident and he had probably been hit by a car but managed to drag himself home and get himself into his basket. He was quite lucky, because he recovered very quickly. I must confess I was pessimistic when I first saw his chest X-ray, and with that swollen head as well, but within 48 hours he seemed to perk up.

Because I had waited a while, the air pockets in his chest had been reabsorbed and he could breathe normally again. I patched up his face and gave him some painkillers and something for the swelling, and then he seemed to be fine.

Simba came back for a check-up a while later and I spoke to a third brother (this one had a full set of teeth), who told me that the cat was now back on the roads, running back and forth. He lived alongside one of the very busy roads between Bath and Frome (where I was working) and he seemed to have this little game he played with cars: he would shoot across the road to see how quick he could be, almost playing 'chicken'. Obviously he had not been quick enough and so he had been hit. Next time, he probably won't be so lucky.

This seems to be a common problem with cats around busy roads. So many of them are not street-wise. Every time I drive along that particular road, cats decide to shoot across when you are really close. Simba was lucky and he is now all right, but that is not always the case.

Bertie, chip in a skip

One day I had a phone call from someone who had found a cat lying in a skip, half unconscious. He brought the cat in for me to check over. He was a really sweet cat, with rather a fat face and lovely symmetrical white markings. He looked very dusty and dirty, as he had been in amongst the rubble in the skip. His front leg had some abrasions and the back leg was sticking out a bit. He was uncomfortable when I was manipulating his leg to find out if there were any fractures or any other serious injuries, but in general he just seemed to be happy to have been picked up from the skip.

The man who found him told me he wanted to keep him if at all possible, if we could not find the owner. When a stray comes into the practice, the procedure is to fill in a form saying where the animal was found, by whom and in what state the animal is. Then you check if it has a microchip that identifies it.

I have seen countless animals coming through the surgery, including a lot of strays, and I have checked hundreds of times for microchips but I have never found any. This time, to my great pleasure and surprise, my scanner read positive on a chip number and I was able to check with the chip company's register. They gave me the owners' name and phone number; I rang the owners and they were thrilled. Bertie the cat had been lost for three days and they thought he was dead. They came to pick him up and I think that the man who found Bertie was rather disappointed, because he wanted to keep him, but obviously it is best for everybody that we found the right owner.

I still did not know what had happened to Bertie and why he had been in a skip. He might have been mistreated by someone, kicked perhaps, or run over. My theory is that he must have been run over by a car and somebody thought he was dead so just dumped him in the skip, but I can only speculate. When I looked at his X-rays I found that he had dislocated his hip: the head of his femur had popped right out of the socket. We popped it back in again under anaesthetic and then sent him home for a long period of cage rest so that the torn tendons had a chance to recover. Next time he came to see me he was in fine form and happily jumped up on to the table.

This little story shows how useful the microchip system can be when your animal goes missing. It also illustrates something else: owners expect their vet to be a brilliant detective! They expect us to be able to work out exactly what has happened in a case like this one. From Bertie's symptoms and injuries it looked to me as if he

TRUDE MOSTUE + **Pets in Practice**

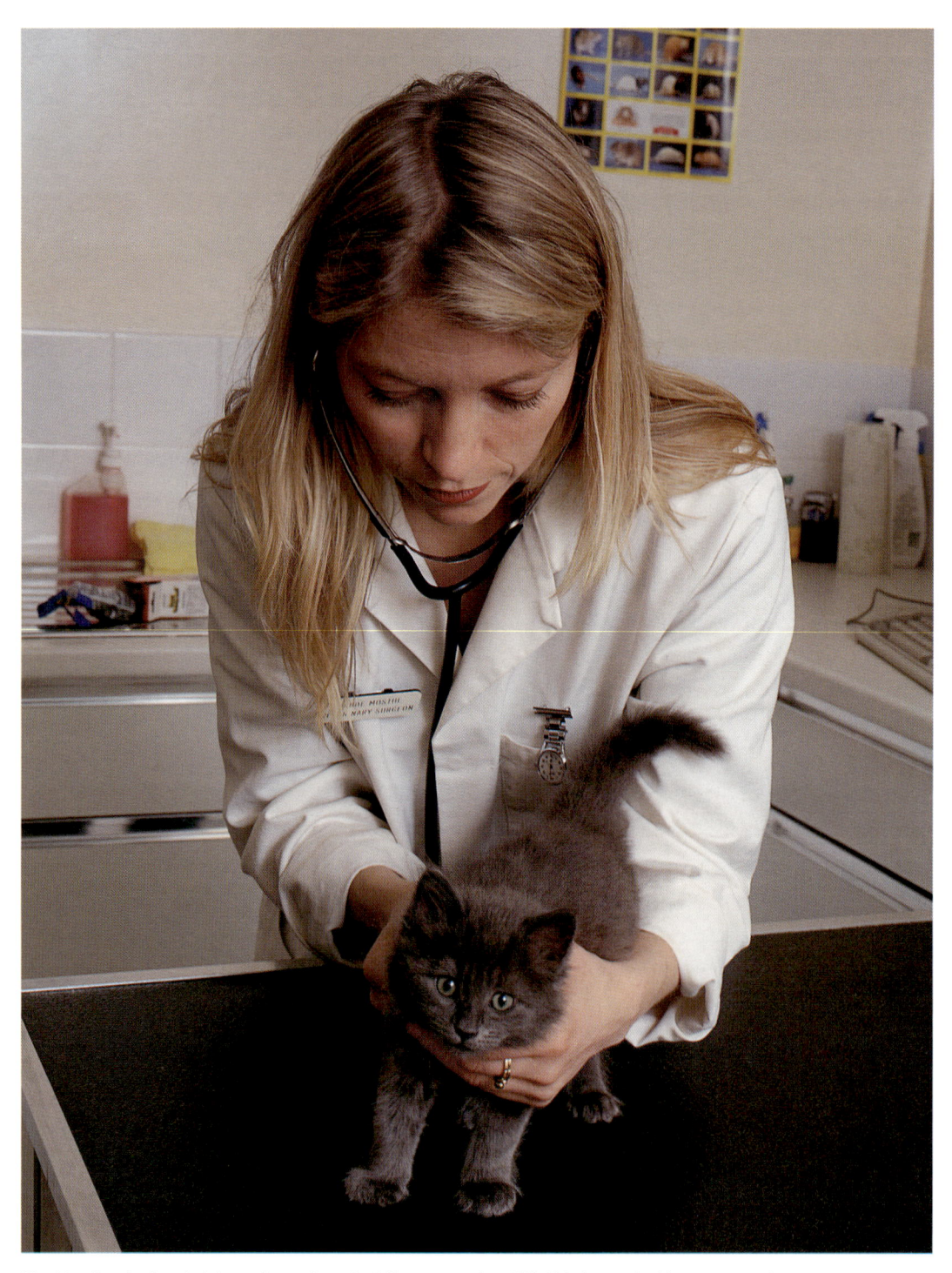

Checking the chest and abdomen is very important if you suspect an RTA. This is me checking my own cat.

had suffered from some form of violence, either by a car or by a person. He already had an old pelvic injury from a previous traffic accident, so maybe he had not learnt the lesson that vehicles can be dangerous.

The bleeding lurcher

I was just finishing off my Saturday surgery and we were closing up when we saw someone running towards the door. There was blood everywhere and they were carrying a dog and I thought: Oh my God, there is something seriously wrong here. I thought the dog must have been hit by a car. The people looked really distressed as we let them in and they were panicking. 'Oh, it's bleeding everywhere, it's bleeding everywhere!' they said.

They were carrying a lurcher, which actually looked fairly happy, sitting comfortably in their arms. When they popped him on my table I just had to jump back – there really was blood absolutely *everywhere*! They were covered in it. 'Where's the blood coming from?' I asked, but they had no idea.

Eventually I discovered that it was coming from the dog's front leg. It had cut itself on some glass on the inside of the leg, where there is a quite big blood vessel, but the blood loss was not at all serious. A very little blood goes a long way and looks much more dramatic than it actually is. The leg was not really bleeding that much – it was not pumping out and there wasn't even a big enough cut to stitch. So I bandaged it up, put a bit of pressure on the wound and then he stopped bleeding and everyone was happy.

Now, if you had been the lurcher's owners, what would you have done in a situation like that? I always say, 'Take it easy.' Once you see that there is some blood

---

Trude's helping hand

Facts about road traffic accidents

- Every year, thousands of dogs and cats are killed in road traffic accidents in the UK.
- The most common road traffic accident injuries are head trauma, fractures, internal bleeding and ruptured diaphragm in cats.

Trude's helping hand

What do to if you find an animal RTA

1. Animals in pain will bite. Use a muzzle, if available, or be very careful when moving the animal.
2. Assess if there is any bleeding that you need to stop, then wrap the animal in a blanket to avoid hurting it more as you lift it.
3. Ring the vet's emergency number to arrange to come into the surgery.
4. Take care of the animal's spine, in case there are any fractures that might worsen if it is twisted or pulled.

coming from somewhere, do not panic. Take it easy. Sit down and try to locate where the blood is coming from. Put anything you can find – your scarf if you are out for a walk, perhaps – around the bleeding site to stop it from bleeding. Carry the animal if necessary and come and see us as soon as possible. It is not a desperate emergency, but if you cannot stop the bleeding and if there is a need to stitch the wound, we need to see the wound as soon as possible. The quicker you get the animal to us, the quicker we can stitch it up. It will cause more trouble if you leave a big cut (for instance, wounds caused by barbed wire) for more than two days than if you bring it straight in, because the wound will have to be debrided. We cannot just stitch it straight back together, because if it is infected and inflamed, we have to snip off the old edges of the wound and then stitch it together again.

In general, cuts on the lower limb and the paw pads look more dramatic than they actually are, because of all the blood. The problem with pads – particularly in dogs, because they are often walked on hard roads – is that it is very difficult to allow the wound to heal. When stitching a cut pad, you have to make sure that no pressure is put on that limb until it is completely healed. This is quite difficult with an active dog. So you have to put on quite a big bandage, which is out of proportion to the seriousness of the injury but it does stop the dog from putting pressure on the wound while it is healing. Otherwise the cut will keep re-opening itself. The pad is very thick and it needs to be immobilised for quite a long time to have even a chance of healing.

Usually cut injuries and stitch-up injuries are not serious; they look more serious than they really are, mainly because of the blood. So just be sensible about it and use whatever you have to hand to put some pressure on the particular site that is bleeding. Dab it clean if it has a lot of dirt on it but, most importantly, put some pressure on it until you can get to your veterinary surgery.

First aid kit to stop bleeding

- Sterile swabs and cotton wool to wipe the wound clean.

- Sterile water or pevidine for cleaning.

- Sterile bigger swab to cover up the wound after cleaning.

- Elastic bandage to apply pressure on the bleeding point.

- Muzzle or string to protect you from bites if the animal is in pain.

The most frequent paw injuries I see in surgery are when a dog has been walking in the park and trodden on something sharp, such as glass. I also get quite a few working dogs that have jumped on barbed wire. Another paw problem I sometimes see, especially in dogs and rabbits, is abrasions from walking on fresh wet concrete. It is caustic at that stage and very painful to the pads.

Brando's ball

It was a Sunday, during my first year in practice, when a family rang up sounding very agitated. 'Can we come in straight away? Our dog might have swallowed his ball.'

They came in with a German shepherd called Brando. He looked all right; he was not breathing through his mouth or choking, but he was breathing quite heavily and I thought it was possible that something was stuck somewhere. The owner told me that his ball was missing and that it was about the size of an apple. Well, I thought he could not possibly have swallowed a ball that big and it was probably just lost in the garden but I decided to have a look. Having sent the owner home, I put Brando under anaesthetic and as I was trying to pass the tube down his throat I suddenly saw, to my great amazement, this big red ball right at the back of his throat. No wonder he was not mouth-breathing: it blocked the whole area, but left just enough room for him to breathe through his nose with a lot of effort.

The problem was: how to dislodge the ball? I tried to grip it with my fingers but it was made of hard plastic rubber and was all slippery with saliva. I tried with crocodile forceps, but it was too slippery for them as well. While I was thinking what to do next, I was feeling under his jaw to see how far down the throat it was and I squeezed the larynx. The ball suddenly shot out and hit me on the forehead, then bounced on to the floor. That was a great relief for both of us! Brando went home with his ball in a plastic bag with strict instructions to buy a larger ball to play with.

Another dog came in to see me with a sharp stick in his throat. He must have run on to the stick with a lot of force: it was about 20–30 cm long and had actually speared the soft tissue beside his windpipe. Luckily I was able to pull it out. Stick injuries like this are very common. Bear that in mind when you are playing with your dog, try to throw big and soft balls instead.

TRUDE MOSTUE + **Pets in Practice**

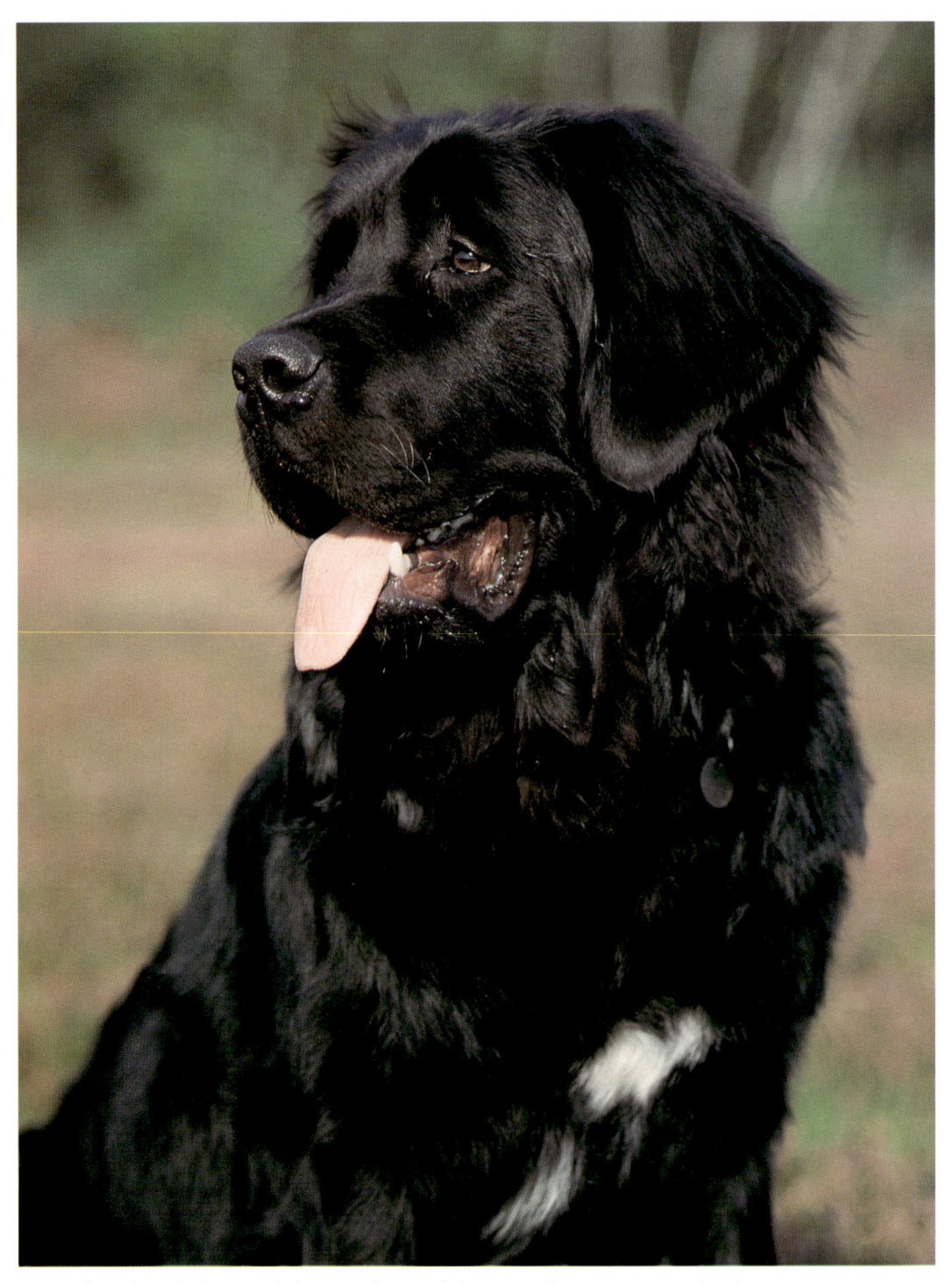

Newfoundland dogs, like Harry, can be huge: but they usually have fantastic temperaments and make good pets.

Harry the Newfoundland

During my first year in practice I was called out at four o'clock in the morning to see Harry, a great big Newfoundland dog weighing about 80 kilos who had a very blown-up stomach. This lovely dog was owned by two really fragile-looking elderly people and I can hardly believe just how much we all went through for Harry. His problem was gastric dilatation/volvulus syndrome (GDV), which means a blown-up and twisted stomach. It is quite common in big deep-chested breeds, but sometimes occurs in smaller breeds. It is serious and you must act immediately when you recognise the symptoms. If the dog recovers, the problem is likely to recur and this is what happened with Harry.

Eventually we had to open up his abdomen and fix his stomach in position so that it could not twist again. Harry managed to come through the surgery and in fact he would have two more dilatations before it was decided that enough was enough.

Some people call it bloat, but that is different from gastric dilatation syndrome. Some dogs have gastric dilation where using a stomach tube to relieve the pressure is enough – while others have a dilation and a twisted stomach which requires surgical attention. The stomach is bloated in GDV but, worse, it twists itself and traps the gas that is forming inside. The dog often goes into shock and can die from heart failure. The mortality rate from gastric dilatation (GVD) is quite high.

The most important symptom you should look out for is when the dog attempts to vomit but does not produce any vomit at all; constant gagging and retching is a very bad sign. The most forward part of the abdomen will feel quite hard and tense. The dog will usually be hunched up and very uncomfortable and restless. Diarrhoea is not usually associated with this problem; it is mainly non-productive vomiting and lethargy.

Gastric dilatation is a true emergency and you should ring the vet immediately to have it checked out, no matter what time of day or night. It needs to be taken very seriously. If it is confirmed, the dog will have to go into hospital and the first priority is to deflate the pressure in the stomach. The surgery mortality rate is high; some do survive but quite a lot will die.

To try to reduce the risk, never feed very large meals and do not take your dog for a run immediately before or after a meal – that is believed to be a trigger for it. We do not really know exactly what causes the condition and so it is difficult to know how to avoid it.

Trude's helping hand

Emergencies: when to worry

Sometimes you do need to worry and really should contact your vet if you notice that any of the following things are happening.

- You see fresh blood in diarrhoea or vomit.
- There is vomit and diarrhoea together and the animal is lethargic.
- A fit lasts for more than about 20 seconds.
- An eyeball is pushed out (prolapsed eye).
- Your pet is choking.
- Your pet has been scalded or burnt.
- Your pet has been stung in the mouth or throat, or has been bitten by an adder.
- The weather is hot and your pet is distressed or seems to have collapsed.
- Your pet is losing or gaining weight quickly.
- Your dog or cat's mouth smells awful (halitosis) and they seem to prefer soft food to hard food.
- Your pet is scratching all the time and you see scabs and raw red areas on the skin.
- Your pet's eye is suddenly closed tight and inflamed.
- Your bitch, who has not been spayed, has a vaginal discharge when she is not meant to be in season.
- Your old dog starts to pant more than it used to when you go for walks and lags behind, and its tongue goes blue when it has some exercise.
- Your cat's belly suddenly looks bloated and the rest of its body is thin.
- Your pet starts to drink excessively and hence urinates more frequently than usual.
- The frequency of urination increases, the animal strains to urinate and you see blood in the urine.
- Your guinea pig stops eating!
- Your dog or cat stops eating and seems to be generally unwell.
- Your dog is suddenly sick and has convulsions after a walk.
- Your dog, after eating a meal, tries to vomit but nothing comes up and it becomes subdued and has a bloated stomach.
- Your tom cat (Persians seem to be predisposed) strains to urinate but nothing comes out.
- Your dog or cat still seems to have diarrhoea after you have starved it for 24 hours and then given it chicken and rice.
- Your animal has been outside and is gagging, followed by excessive salivation.
- Your cage bird has stopped eating and its feathers are all fluffed up.
- Your rat has a bloody discharge from its nostrils and loses weight.
- Your kitten's eyes have a discharge and it sneezes a lot.
- Your hamster has lots of scabs on its skin and loses weight.

Puffy

Puffy was the nickname I gave him, for obvious reasons. He was a Weimeraner puppy but when he came in to see me his whole head was swollen up like a big ball and he looked more like a shar-pei, with just little slits for eyes. He couldn't even see me and he just sat there groaning to himself.

He had been stung by something on the side of his cheek. Actually it looked worse than it really was. I gave him some antihistamines and when he came back the next day I did not recognise him: he was a nice slim-faced Weimeraner again!

We quite often see animals that have been stung in the summer. In another case, a golden retriever was brought in with a hugely swollen throat. Even with all that thick retriever coat I could see this massive lump and he seemed to have no neck at all – just a continuous swelling from his chin to his chest. He had been scratching furiously at his neck and the skin was all red raw. At first I thought he had a huge cyst, but when I looked more closely I found two small puncture wounds. I still do not know what had bitten him, but antihistamines and antibiotics did the trick.

Trude's helping hand

Home first aid

- **Burns**: Cool immediately with cold water and contact the vet. In the meantime, cover with moist sterile dressing or clingfilm and reassure the animal, keeping calm yourself and keeping the pet quiet.

- **Sprains and strains**: Use a cold-water compress to reduce swelling and pain.

- **Stings**: If a sting is in the mouth or throat it could swell up and restrict breathing so get to the vet quickly. Also go to the vet if the sting is in the eye, ear or anus. Otherwise use home remedies – even a simple cold-water compress will help to reduce pain and swelling, and rubbing with half a freshly cut onion can help as well.
  - Bee stings: Remove sting very carefully to make sure you get the whole sting out and don't in the meantime squeeze more venom in. Apply an alkaline substance, e.g. bicarbonate of soda.
  - Wasp stings: Apply an acid, e.g. vinegar.

- **Adder bites**: Keep calm, and keep the animal calm, but get veterinary help immediately. If you know what you are doing, apply a tourniquet to prevent the poison spreading, but only for a short while. Carry the animal to the nearest telephone – do not let it walk as this would encourage the poison to spread.

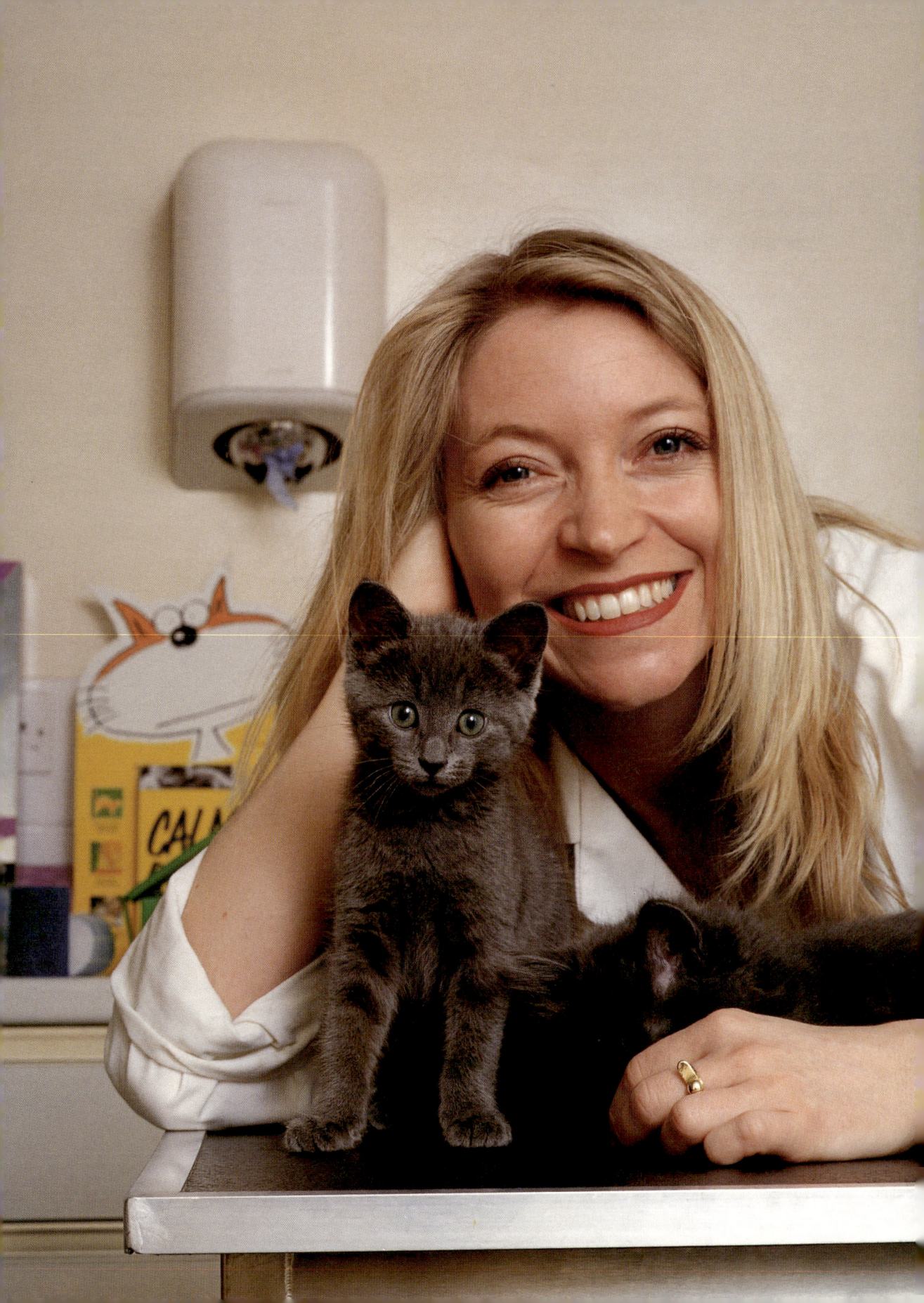

CHAPTER 3
BREEDS AND BREEDING
– OR NOT

Some pet owners intentionally breed from their animals but many more find themselves with puppies, kittens, baby rabbits and so on quite by mistake and then have difficulty in finding homes for them all. With so many thousands or even millions of unwanted baby animals having to be destroyed, I want to tell you some stories about why and how pets can be neutered so that these mistakes do not happen in the first place and to point out that neutering also prevents quite a few other problems, both physical and behavioural. Then I want to talk about some of the different breeds – some of which have serious genetic problems – and what you should look out for when you are choosing a new pet and also that the best pedigree cat or dog is not necessarily the most healthy animal.

Harvey, the Westie with attitude

West Highland white terrier puppies are always very cute and sweet, but most people do not realise that what they are buying is what I consider to be a big Rottweiler in disguise. In my experience, a Westie's temperament and personality are more those of a large dog than of a small dog, which makes me admire them but it also means that they are more determined to get what they want and do what they want – especially the males – like all terriers.

I first met a Westie called Harvey when he was a little eight-week-old puppy and of course he was really sweet, as they all are. He wanted his vaccines ... no, that is not true: I am sure *he* did not want his vaccines, but his owners wanted him to be inoculated when he was eight weeks old and again when he was 12 weeks old.

As you can see from this picture kittens, and puppies, are lovely. But, too many of them are born unnecessarily, cannot find homes and have to be put down.

As most Westie puppies do, he squealed his head off when I gave him his first vaccination. As always, I felt like Cruella de Ville, and I could see from the look on his face that he thought I really was the witch from somewhere unpleasant. Whenever puppies squeal when you vaccinate them you always feel bad, because their owners already feel bad about bringing them in and they are very protective about their little puppies.

Anyway, Harvey came to see me when he was eight weeks old, got his vaccination and went home again. Then he came back when he was 12 weeks old, got his second jabs and squealed even more, because now he knew for sure that I was a vicious person, he knew that he was not going to like me and he knew that this was going to be a place he was going to hate in the future. Unfortunately, most Westies do spend a lot of their time at the vet's because the breed is prone to skin problems and allergies and they come and go all the time.

When Harvey came back that second time and after he had squealed his head off, the owners and I started to talk about behaviour. Usually I spend some time with puppy owners talking about training, insurance, worming and all the preventive measures, and also about teeth, hygiene and so on – things that are important to know when getting a puppy, particularly if it is your first dog.

Harvey was owned by a couple and I suspect that he was a child substitute for them. They were really protective about him and seemed to feel quite bad about doing him any harm, even though it was for his own good. They just wanted the best for him. Sometimes the tendency to overprotect animals and treat them too much like little human beings gives them a lot of attitude – and Harvey already had a lot of attitude by the time he was 12 weeks old. He tried to bite me when I touched him and it was not the kind of friendly play bite that most puppies give.

So we talked about behaviour and training classes and it soon became obvious that the couple had something to say, something they did not really want to tell me. Finally they came out with it. They were getting quite concerned because he had already started to hang on to their legs and was beginning to be a permanent fixture around their ankles, forever trying to mate with their trousers or their slippers. He was still much too young to be castrated and so I advised them to be patient, and in the meantime to go to training classes and socialise him. I also suggested that they should regularly handle his ears, his mouth, his feet and so on, so that it would be easier for me when they next came to the surgery. I asked them to come back when he was about six or seven months old.

Five months passed and Harvey came back to see me. By that time his owners were quite distressed. The poor postman had become quite used to having Harvey hanging on to his leg while he was delivering their letters, and they told me that Harvey had such a high sex drive that he had even been trying it on with the neighbour's rabbits – which naturally upset the neighbour's children, especially as Harvey tended to dig holes through the hedge and jump on to the rabbits while they were eating their food with their backs to him.

I could not help laughing and the owners thought it was quite funny as well, but it was becoming a nuisance, particularly if they were having parties or when people came to see them. Yes, it can sound funny if you do not experience it, but the joke wears thin when you have to live with it.

There seemed to be no stopping him. For instance, they had been to a London café where they could sit outside; Harvey was with them and had spotted a ponyskin handbag at another table. He launched himself across to the other table, grabbed hold of the bag and tried to do his business. The bag was quite expensive and its owner was none too pleased, as you can imagine.

Harvey's owners had had enough and he was admitted for castration, which went quite well. We made sure that everything else was fine with him but discovered that he still had one of his baby teeth, so I took that one out to give some space for the new teeth.

After the operation it was about two or three months before he started to calm down but, slowly, he began to redirect his attention from legs and fluffy objects to food. That is what sometimes happens when dogs have been neutered. They switch their energy to something else, which all too often is food. The last news I heard about Harvey was that he was attending the weight watchers' clinic at my old practice.

Neutering dogs is more and more common and most male dogs are now castrated. They do not have to be and I often advise people to wait and see. If the dog becomes really frisky and starts to roam and run after the girls, then I suggest he should be brought in as soon as possible, mainly for his own safety. When dogs roam and try to find bitches on heat, they usually roam across the streets on their adventures and that is when they are hit by a car. Most canine road traffic accidents involve males on their searches for bitches and so it is probably safer to stop them from roaming by castrating them.

Penny

Penny, a little Jack Russell terrier, was about 10 years old when she came in with pyometra, an infection of the womb in unspayed bitches.

It was quite easy to diagnose pyometra because she was discharging from the vulva and she was very lethargic. Her blood count showed a very high proportion of white blood cells, indicating to me that there was highly aggressive infection in her body. X-rays showed a big uterus filling up her abdomen.

Penny was really ill with it but she was only 10 years old (which is not too old for a Jack Russell Terrier) and her owner wanted to give her a go. So we operated on her and it went well, but it was touch and go because her uterus was so big and there is a danger of rupturing the uterus when you are handling it in the abdomen. It is a tricky and dangerous operation. If you are lucky, they get through it, but you can equally well be unlucky and lose them.

When I had told the owner that Penny had pyometra, I was suprised that she said, 'Oh well, I knew, because I've lost two other bitches to the same trouble.' I have come across that situation so many times. Even if they are breeding bitches, you can spay them once you stop breeding from them, and most people don't breed from them after a certain age.

I find it really frustrating to speak to people who do not realise that unspayed bitches are prone to pyometra or, even worse, those who *do* know. If you lose another bitch from the same condition and you know that you could have prevented it, why do you do it? If it is a question of money, it will be more expensive in the long run to pay for a pyometra operation: when they are operated on for pyometra you have to spay them anyway, and also they are then at a higher risk of dying because they are already ill when you are operating.

Neutering bitches helps to prevent not only pyometra, but also mammary tumours. It has been proved, scientifically, that 'entire' bitches are more prone to mammary carcinomas than spayed bitches. These cancerous tumours are usually malignant and they do spread to other organs if they are not caught in time. I have seen many different cases with mammary carcinomas and, again, the majority of the owners tell me that their previous bitch had the same thing. It amazes me. Why do they let a second bitch go the same way as the last one when they know the risk? It makes no sense!

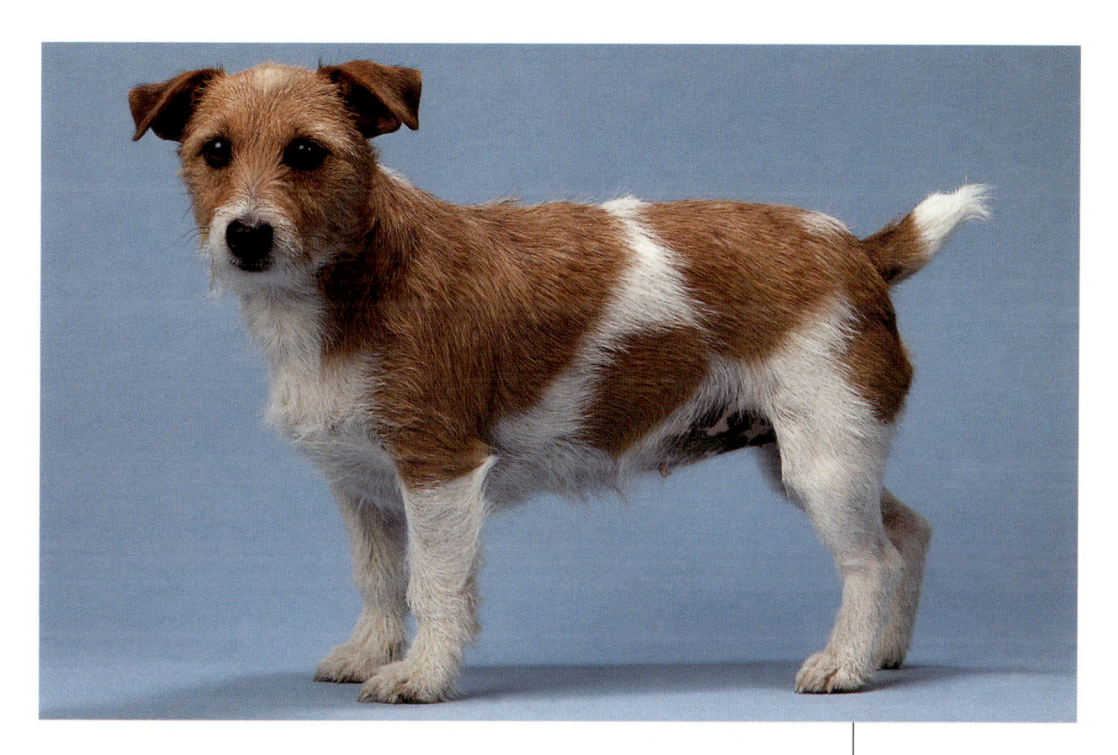

At college we were taught that if you spay a bitch between her first and second season, you decrease the risk of mammary carcinomas, though you do not take it away completely. It is the same principle with people: you do not take the risk away completely but you do decrease it.

Spaying bitches still has plenty of advantages. I know there is a lot of controversy around the subject of spaying at present but I normally explain the pros and cons to my clients and then it is up to them to make the decision. I understand if they choose not to do it and I understand if they choose to do it. All I can say is that at least you know the spayed bitch will not get pyometra, that she will not run some of the risks of pregnancy (such as having a caesarian or other difficulties while giving birth), that there will fewer unwanted puppies (there are quite enough of them around already) and that there is less risk of developing uterine carcinomas.

Jack Russell terriers are lovely dogs. They are friendly and loyal – sometimes too loyal to their owners at the expense of strangers.

Making a decision about neutering in general, whether for dogs or cats and males or females, is harder than most people realise, because it is elective surgery. Should it go wrong (because you know that, statistically, some animals will react badly to an anaesthetic) and they die, you feel terrible as you know that you have opted to subject a healthy animal to an operation. It is not a life-saving operation and it does carry a risk (all General Anaesthetic's do), so a lot of guilt is involved.

Losing animals because of the anaesthetic when they are being neutered is a vet's worst nightmare. It is a risk that has to be taken and fortunately such deaths are very rare, but we emphasise to owners when we take animals in that there is always an anaesthetic risk. Then again, there is always a risk even crossing the street. You are more likely to be hit by a car and killed than to die from an anaesthetic.

Neutering cats

In contrast to these emergency operations, the neutering of cats is usually more routine. In fact, there are so few unneutered cats these days that I have never seen a pyometra case in a cat in England. I saw a lot of it in Norway, though, because the neutering policy there is slacker than it is in this country (I suppose there are fewer cats). British people seem to be more aware of the problem of unwanted cats and they are responsible enough to have their animals neutered.

To spay cats we make a small cut on the side, through which we remove the whole uterus. The cat goes home with a few stitches in her side and the operation is usually without complications.

In the case of a family cat, the queen should be spayed at between five and six months of age. But be warned that in the spring cats seem to come into season even when they are as young as four months of age – basically because cats depend on the length of daylight to be stimulated to come into season, which is why cats are calling in the spring. So do not be fooled: if your cat is around four months old in March or April, or even in February, she is quite capable of becoming pregnant if an appropriate tom is hanging around.

Most tom cats are castrated these days as well. Very few people are prepared to put up with the smell and behaviour of an unneutered tom cat. They certainly will smell – the urine smells really strongly – and they will spray, because they have extremely strong sexual territorial behaviour.

Toms rarely come into the surgery but when they do they are full of abscesses because they fight so often. As they get older it is quite sad because they keep on losing their fights and so are covered with wounds and abscesses, and if they are not attended to they would probably die of septicaemia.

I have argued with quite a few male clients who want to keep toms entire, but I do not think it is fair on the animal when it is suffering so much from injuries throughout the time when it is entire. Also a lot of toms come in as road traffic accidents because they roam all over the place in search of a calling queen. So I do recommend the castration of cats as well as dogs. It is more social (they are very antisocial when they are not castrated) and it is a very simple operation.

Pretty little Tilly

A lovely little albino ferret called Tilly came in to see me with her owner, who was worried because she had heard that jills (female ferrets) can die if they are not spayed.

I agreed with her that this was a potential danger and explained why. Jills will remain in season until they are mated. Now, in the wild, that is not a problem – they will mate almost as soon as they come into season in the spring and they will become pregnant. Domesticated ferrets do not always have the opportunity of mating, and in that case a jill faces the problem of being in season continuously for perhaps six months, so that she is under the influence of oestrogen for much longer than normal. Too much oestrogen can suppress the production of red blood cells in the bone marrow, hence causing anaemia; the poor little ferret loses her appetite, gets depressed and dehydrated and eventually develops a fever and might die. Even if the situation does not go that far, her vulva will remain swollen and exposed throughout the breeding season if she is unmated, and so infection is likely to find its way into her womb.

We decided that the best answer was to spay Tilly and I booked her in for the operation a week later. We also agreed that she might be happier with a male companion and that we should castrate him.

I find ferrets are notoriously tricky to anaesthetise and when I put Tilly under general anaesthetic she stopped breathing just as I was about to cut the skin. It was very difficult to get the right balance – to make the anaesthesia deep enough to operate without the risk of stopping her breathing. I decided to abandon the operation and rang the owner to explain. The owner was just very relieved that Tilly was all right.

She was a sweet little ferret. Usually I never trust them but with Tilly I felt brave enough to handle her and was tickling her tummy when she came round from the anaesthetic. So now we moved on to plan B, which was to find a boyfriend for her but to vasectomise rather than castrate him. This would mean that he could mate with Tilly and bring her out of season, but without actually making her pregnant. That would get over the problem of prolonged oestrus and the risk of bone marrow disease.

We found her new boyfriend, called Bentley, at Longleat, and there was no problem with the vasectomy. The last I heard, Bentley was being very macho and was dragging poor Tilly around by the scruff of her neck in typical male ferret fashion all the time. I hope that they will settle well together and that he will not bother her too much!

Macho Minky

Minky was a polecat-coloured ferret from Frome. He came in the day after I'd had the experience with Tilly reacting badly to the anaesthetic and so I was a little nervous about Minky, but he was a big, beefy and cheeky hob (male), which made him much less of a risk.

Minky's owner brought him into the surgery on a lead. It surprised some of us but it is not uncommon for ferrets to be taken for walks on a lead. The head nurse was a little wary of Minky and I think we were all slightly worried about him once the owner had gone, because we didn't know him. If you are not used to ferrets, you do worry when they start to nibble on your hand, but Minky was fine.

He was quite a big ferret and had come in to be castrated. Castration in ferrets improves the smell as well as reducing their sexual drive. Sometimes quite an aggressive streak comes with sexual behaviour and so neutering calms them down as well. The owner told me that Minky would get a bit frisky with her cushions in the dining room and on the sofa – in fact he was trying to mount anything that moved and anything that didn't. So ferrets are not that different from dogs!

I chose to give Minky a slightly different anaesthetic than I had given to Tilly the day before and he was fine. The main problem was how to hold him for an injection. Ferrets are quite hard to hold and handle, unless you know exactly what you are doing. It is like trying to restrain a long wriggling sausage with teeth at one end and four sets of small sharp claws, but once you have stabilised the head you are fine. It was quite hilarious trying to inject him: I had three or four nurses, each holding one part of him while I was holding out this fat little hind leg and looking for a tiny short muscle to inject. But in the end, I am pleased to say, the anaesthetic went well and the operation itself went well.

When I saw Minky a couple of weeks later to take his stitches out, I spoke more to his very sweet owner: she was devoted to Minky but was looking forward to him being less smelly. Those who keep ferrets get used to the smell – it is other people who notice it, which is just the same with dogs. I do not mind the mustiness of a ferret as long as it is not too strong.

Minky on the table with George the nurse. George is preparing Minky for the operation. The bubble wrap is used to prevent heat loss during surgery.

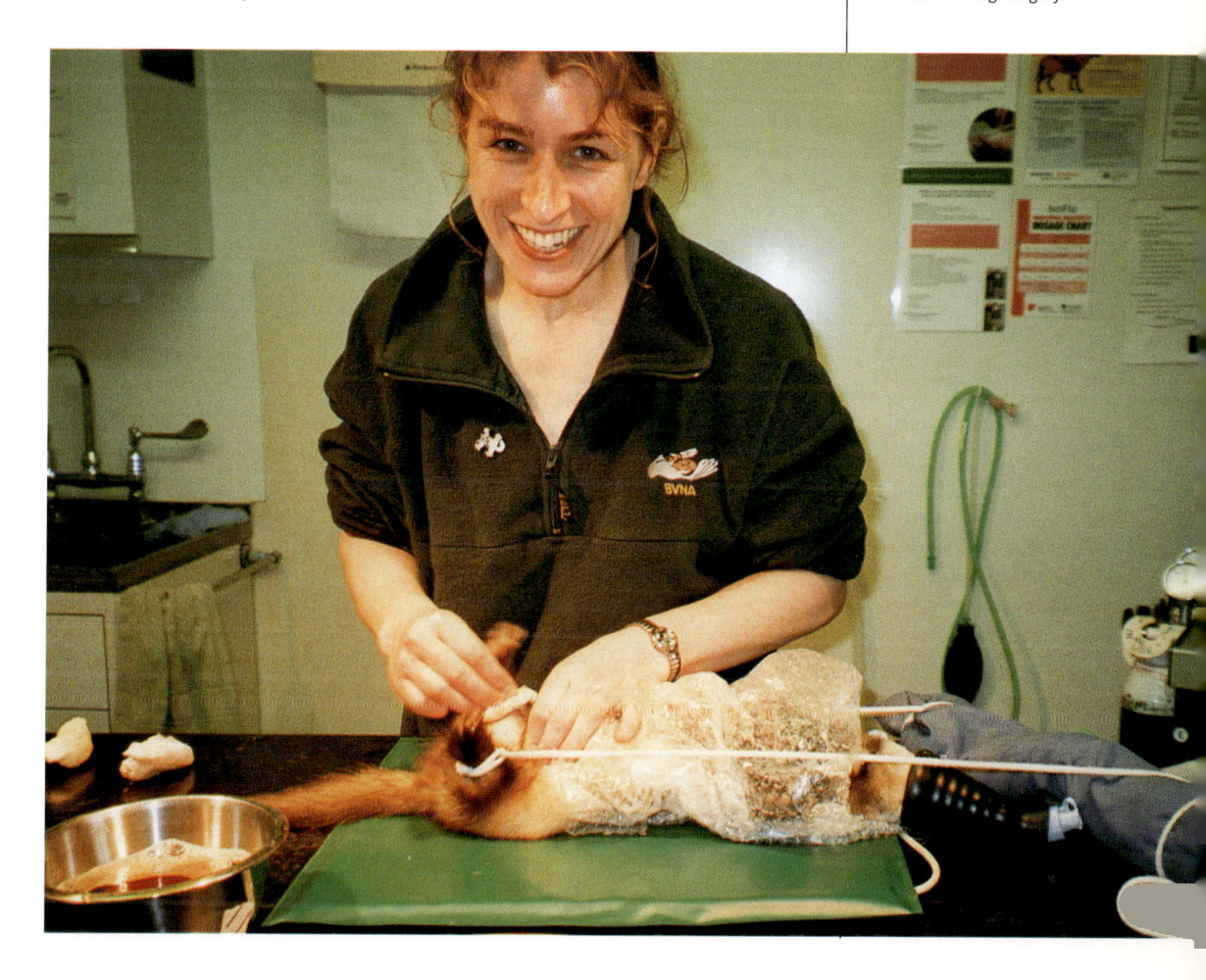

Pregnancy

Most bitches reach sexual maturity when they are between six and 20 months old, and cats between seven and 12 months old (or even younger, as already mentioned). So start to watch out in case there are roving dogs and toms in the area. Bitches come 'on heat' or 'in season' (i.e. ready to mate) twice a year and you can tell when she is ready because you will notice a few drops of blood from her vulva for two or three days. About 10 or 12 days later she is at peak fertility (ovulation) and that is the ideal time for her to breed – if that is what you really want (think hard about this).

Queens are very obvious when they are in season: their behaviour announces it to the whole wide world, especially if they are not mated. A Siamese, for example, has a special mating voice and will shout for a mate so loudly and persistently that even the dimmest owner will know what she is on about. Queens also adopt a different posture, which again any owner will soon recognise – bottom in the air, tail up!

The length or term of a pregnancy, if you calculate from when a bitch was first mated, can be anything from about 56 to 72 days (shorter in smaller breeds and longer in large ones). The trouble is, if there has been more than one mating you do not necessarily know when conception actually took place. With queens, the average is 65 to 67 days, but again it can be anything from about 56 to 70 days.

If you think that your pet might be pregnant, you can ask the vet to confirm it and give you an idea of when the birth is likely to be. The vet can also give you advice about diet, exercise and good places for the birth. Then you can prepare yourself and your pet for the big day.

Giving birth

Vets (and doctors) always like long words and so they call giving birth 'parturition', which literally means 'bringing forth'. They also have a word for difficult births: 'dystocia', which is a combination of two Greek terms for 'ill' and 'birth'.

Dystocia is when a pregnant animal cannot push the foetus through the birth canal without assistance and quite often this is because of the breed – for example, dog breeds with big or squashed heads (e.g. pekingese or bulldog), or breeds that are prone to uterine inertia (inability to strain, e.g. dachshund), or the puppies are too big (e.g. corgi, or when there are only one or two puppies) – or because the mum is too fat or rather old, or even because the babies are too small or too few to stimulate the necessary contractions. But there might also be an obstruction of some kind in the birth canal, including babies that are too big or are already dead. Usually dystocia means that the mother will have to undergo a caesarean section in the surgery, and if a birth is obviously not going according to plan, you need to contact your vet as soon as possible for help.

Most animals, if they are fit and healthy, give birth easily without any help at all and often prefer to do so when you are not there. Indeed, some of them seem to cross their legs and wait until you have gone for a cup of tea, and when you get back there they are with little squirming babies, looking smug. With some pedigree dogs there just might be problems and you need to be aware of them but for heaven's sake do not start fussing about. If *you* seem to be worried, then your bitch will be as well and she really does not need the extra stress, thanks very much!

Cats almost never have problems giving birth, nor do rabbits. With the various small mammals in cages, you do need to leave them alone to get on with it, as many of them are liable to kill their own young if you interfere in any way. That is a perfectly natural reaction of any wild animal that thinks its litter has been discovered by a predator, even if your pet knows perfectly well that you do not count as one.

Breeds

Once upon a time, as they say, all dogs looked much the same, because they were wolves. But people began to choose different things about

Trude's helping hand

Facts about neutering

- Why are pets neutered?
  - To prevent roaming and hypersexuality in dogs.
  - To prevent pregnancy, pyometra and mammary carcinomas in bitches.
  - To prevent uterine carcinomas and improve temper in rabbits.
  - To prevent bone marrow disease in female ferrets and reduce smelliness in male ferrets.
  - To avoid unwanted puppies, kittens and baby rabbits being born.

- Male dogs are neutered at the age of six to seven months.

- Bitches are generally spayed between their first and second season, but some practices spay before the first season. Ask your vets which policy they prefer.

- Queens are usually spayed at five or six months old.

- Have a look in the rescue centres and see how many older animals need a new home:
  - There are 6.7m dogs in the UK.
  - There are hundreds of dogs in rescue homes.
  - Every year thousands of dogs are put to sleep because homes cannot be found for them.

TRUDE MOSTUE + Pets in Practice

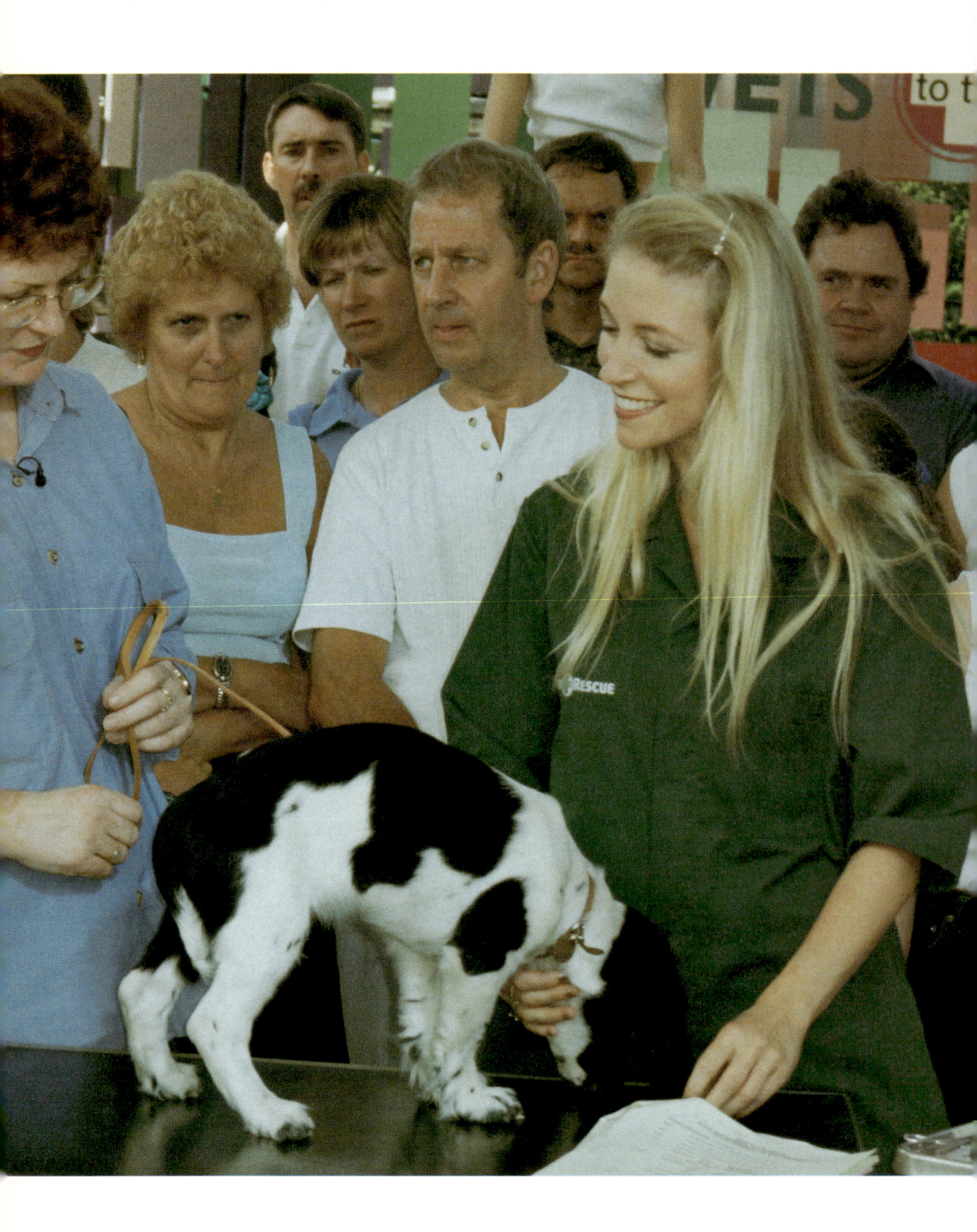

dogs that they wanted to encourage to make them useful and gradually those differences turned into breeds. For most of the 15,000-year history of the dog, the breeding has been thoroughly practical – people chose dogs for specific work, such as rounding up sheep and cattle, hunting for the table or for sport, fighting, guarding, rescuing, going to war, pulling sledges and carts and carrying burdens. Dogs had a sense of purpose and were necessary; they were true working partners.

But then, in very recent times, people began to breed dogs more for their looks than their working ability, like long dangly ears or fancy coats. Others bred dogs smaller and smaller so that they became almost like toys: you could pick them up easily, which gave you more control over them. One trouble with small dogs is that they do not *know* they are small dogs: inside they feel just the same as a big dog 10 times their size, and that can get them into all sorts of difficulties.

Today most people breed a certain type of dog just because they happen to like that type of dog, though some are still bred to work. It is often the working breeds that cause the most problems to owners who do not use them for work – the poor dog does not really know what to do with itself now that it no longer has a proper role in life!

It is not only the size and coat and ears that have changed since the dog was a wolf. Very often the type of work the dog was bred for has developed its temperament and sometimes its shape. For example, obviously a dog like a Dobermann has the instinct to guard and probably to attack intruders, and it is large and muscular to carry out its job. A greyhound is built for speed and has the instinct to chase a prey that it can see (which is why it is sometimes called a gaze-hound) whereas a bloodhound is bred to track its target by using its nose rather than its eyes and to do so for mile after mile with dogged determination – it needs stamina rather than speed.

In several breeds the change of shape has gone much too far, especially during the twentieth century. When you look at the grossly squashed faces of bulldogs that can hardly breathe, it is hard to imagine that originally they could grip a bull by the nose and hang on in there for major bull-baiting events in big arenas. When you look at some of the dachshunds, it is hard to believe that they were originally bred as hunting dogs. And when you look at a toy poodle, all pampered and primped and puffed and pompommed, can you imagine that it is at heart a highly

I am often asked to judge at dog shows, and I always enjoy seeing dogs in such good condition.

intelligent serious hunter's dog that was used to retrieve waterfowl from the marshes? Or that a little Pomeranian once used to be a sheepdog?

Lots of people like mongrels and moggies – dogs and cats of no particular breed but with plenty of character. The main advantage of going for a proper breed, especially if you are buying a puppy or kitten, is that (in theory) you have a pretty good idea of what they are going to look like and know quite a lot about what their character will be. For example, a terrier behaves very differently from a labrador, as well as looking very different.

Trude's helping hand

Stages of giving birth

Before parturition starts in bitches and queens, you might see some of the following signs that it is about to happen.

- The tummy gets bigger as the pregnancy progresses, especially during the second half of the term. It is usually very round just before the birth in a queen, but tends to change from round to pear-shaped in a bitch in the final week.

- The mammary glands are more obvious in the last few days, or in the last two to three weeks for a first-time bitch; they become pink in queens in the last two to three weeks.

- Bitches often seem to be more docile and quieter than usual during pregnancy.

- The mother makes a nest and wants to be alone. She might hide somewhere, especially if she is a cat (who usually decides for herself where to nest, whatever other lovely places you might have offered her).

- She goes off her food.

- Her vaginal lips get swollen and flabby.

- Her temperature drops quite sharply within 24 hours before giving birth, especially if she is a bitch and especially if she is a small breed.

- She has colostrum in her teats.

All of this is part of the preparation stage. *The signs and activities of the normal labour stages for bitches and queens after that are as follows.*

- First-stage labour (up to 12 hours but often much longer for first-time mothers): restlessness; nest-making; onset of contractions; panting; possibly shivering because of temperature drop; sometimes vomiting; queens might meow and groom themselves.

- Second-stage labour (three to 12 hours): straining starts – more co-ordinated contractions; mother may be standing, lying on side or crouching; waterbag for the first baby starts to appear and the mother might bite at it or it might rupture by itself, releasing fluid; first puppy or kitten pops out in its amniotic sac;

Among dogs, there are so many breeds that there is almost bound to be something for everybody, whether you want a big dog or a small one, a dog that needs lots of exercise or one that needs very little, a dog for a small flat in a city or a dog for the great outdoors, a dog that looks pretty but needs plenty of grooming (which some people enjoy) or one that more or less keeps its own coat in good order, a dog that does not moult hairs on your carpet, a lap dog or not, and so on. The important thing is to get a breed that suits your own lifestyle and your own character – that way you have a better chance of a successful

mother opens the sac by licking it vigorously and usually chews the umbilical cord to break it. (If the mother fails to release the baby from its amniotic sac, quickly do it yourself.)

- Third-stage labour: more contractions; placentas expelled alternately with birth of other foetuses (which usually come out much quicker than the first one). Mother normally eats the placentas. Usually, with a bitch, the first puppy takes about 15 to 60 minutes to be born, then there is another 15 minutes before the placenta is expelled, then a rest for half an hour to an hour or so before the next bout of straining for the second puppy, but this varies (sometimes puppies come out in quick succession, sometimes there can be an hour or more between each puppy); average time to deliver four to eight puppies is about six hours, maximum time about 12 hours. Production of discharge called uteroverdin (greenish-brown in bitch, reddish-brown in queen) is normal.
- After the birth: mother cleans up the litter and herself; young start to suckle. With a lot of puppies, she will lose a lot of calcium through her milk so watch out for signs of calcium deficiency (trembling and shaking, for example); the vet can give calcium intravenously if the deficiency is bad.

When to seek veterinary help:

- There is no sign of labour at the end of the pregnancy term.
- More than 30 minutes pass between first signs of the waterbag and birth of the first baby.
- The mother has been straining unproductively for more than an hour.
- One or two puppies have been born and the bitch is straining and straining but no more puppies appear.
- She seems to be getting weak from straining.
- No foetuses are born but there is a reddish or green discharge.
- She has been in second-stage labour for more than 12 hours.

partnership though, of course, there are no guarantees. In the end, most people choose an animal simply because they like it, whatever it is.

There is also quite a wide range to choose from in cat breeds, though they were never bred for 'work': all cats hunt anyway, and can you imagine breeding a cat to pull a sledge, or bring back a pheasant that has just been shot, or rescue people from under an avalanche or track down a criminal? I can just see a cat looking at you with disbelief and saying, 'Who, *me*? Do *what*? You must be joking! Tell the dog to do it.'

In cats, the breed differences are not nearly so varied as in dogs. You do not get the equivalent of a Great Dane cat or a chihuahua cat, after all, but you can get different colours and coat patterns, different types of coat and even different characters. For example, they say that Siamese and Burmese cats are more like dogs than cats, and both of them are very talkative with people.

Several cat breeds have their own special problems, especially those with long hair, and you need to be aware of the problems before you decide to get one. Persians look very pretty with their long, fine hair but that hair easily gets tangled up into impossible mats if you do not groom it daily; also many Persians have been bred with very squashed noses and, like bulldogs, they can suffer from breathing problems. Naturally, if I wanted fluff I would prefer a Norwegian Forest cat to a Persian – it looks very like a Maine Coon cat and can be just as big (more than 7 kg in some cases) with a 'double' semi-longhair coat, very fluffy underneath, and a proper cat-shaped head. But then again I am a vet and will always try to avoid potentially unhealthy animals to get away from work!

You need to think twice about a Manx cat (the one born with no tail) because the gene that gives it no tail often also causes spinal problems. And I do not think I would go for a Scottish Fold, whose main feature is ears that are folded over, or a Munchkin which has stunted legs like a dachshund. Why on earth do people breed deformities like that?

You can also get different 'breeds' in some of the small cage mammals. For example, there are two species of chinchilla to choose from, both from South America, and various colours have been developed since they were first bred in captivity in the 1920s for their fur. As for guinea pigs, there are three breeds – the English with short fine hair, the Abyssinian with rough wiry hair and the very long-haired Peruvian –

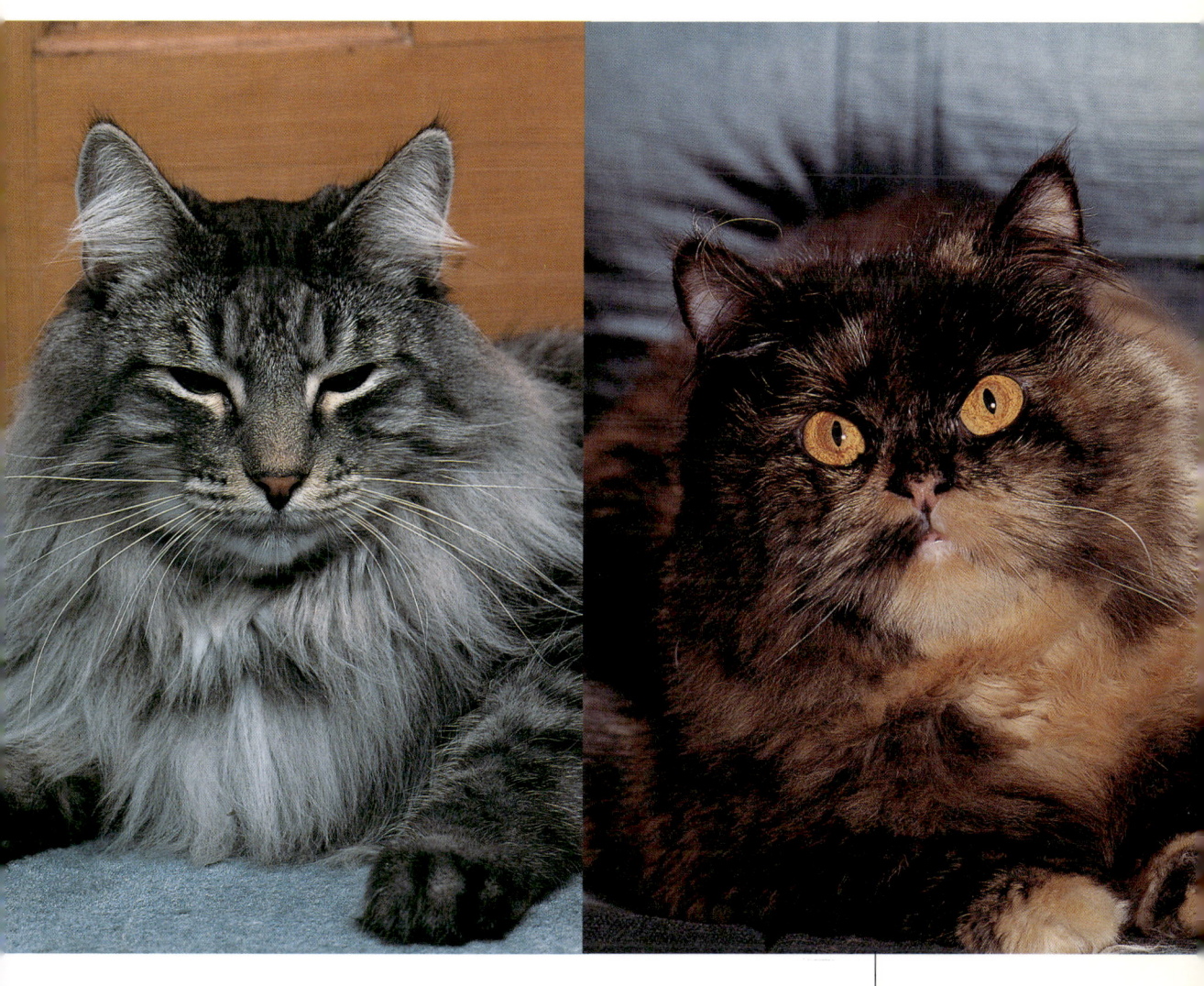

and in all of them you have a wide choice of colours and coat patterns. With hamsters, there are several different species but in Britain most of them are the Syrian or golden hamster.

Rabbits can be fancy breeds or fur breeds, and various divisions in each group. With the fancy rabbits you get quite a range of size and shape as well as coat colour: the great big Flemish can weigh more than 8 kg, which looks ridiculous next to a 1 kg Netherland dwarf rabbit! And you can get rabbits with lop ears or rabbits with upright ears, rabbits with fluffy coats or rabbits with short coats and so on. There are probably about 80 different rabbit breeds to choose from.

Norwegian forest cats (above left) are quite a new 'breed' – and were developed from big, long-haired tabby moggies. That's why it is such a healthy breed!
Persian cats (above) have been specially bred to have long hair and as a result may develop breathing problems.

Pet mice are mostly of one species but in lots of different colours and coat patterns, and you can even get mice with long hair. Rats, too, come in lots of different colours and patterns. Ferrets also come in different colours, though not very many of them: most ferrets are either pink-eyed white albinos or dark-eyed 'polecat' ferrets (they are not actually wild polecats – they just have similar colour and markings), but some people are now breeding different colours and coat patterns.

You don't have breeds among reptiles, just different groups and species. Chelonians are the ones with shells (tortoises, turtles and terrapins); lizards include iguanas, geckos and the like; and of course snakes include everything from a nice little garter snake to a massive boa constrictor. Among the amphibians perhaps the most common pets are newts and salamanders, but I hardly ever see any of those, and even more rarely do I see a pet frog or toad. Then there are pet fish, and here of course the choice is huge, especially among the different tropical species, with all those lovely colours and funny shapes.

With birds, it is usually just a choice of species rather than breed – an African Grey parrot or a Senegal parrot, say – but with budgies you have plenty of colours to choose from.

Choosing a dog

You first need to decide whether you want a pedigree dog or a mongrel. Whichever you go for, its temperament is probably the most important thing.

For a mongrel, contact your local rescue centre – they always have plenty of litters of crossbred puppies. But beware of possible problems; it is likely that nothing at all is known about their vaccination record or medical history.

For a pedigree puppy, contact the Kennel Club or look at dog magazines for breeders' addresses and for advice on breeds. Be aware that breeders are not usually neutral in their opinions, which means you will not necessarily get the breed that is right for you. When choosing a breed, temperament, size and health are more important than looks. Whatever the breed, make sure it has not been mutilated by having its tail docked!

There are several questions you need to ask the breeder before making your decisions on which dog to buy.

TRUDE MOSTUE + Pets in Practice

Trude's helping hand

Buying a pet

Before you even think of buying or 'rescuing' an animal, do your research: go to the library, read pet-keeping magazines, talk to your vet, get advice from the RSPCA and special organisations such as PDSA or the National Canine Defence League or Cats Protection League, and check the internet or even have a chat with your local vet!

- Find out everything you need to know about your pet's needs:
  - Dietary needs
  - How much space it needs
  - What sort of living quarters it needs
  - Natural behaviour
  - How long the species lives on average
  - How much it is likely to cost you in terms of food, veterinary bills and time
  - Whether it is likely to be the right animal for any children you have (from the animal's point of view, that is)
  - Whether it will need to be trained and, if so, how.

- Make sure this type of pet's routines will fit in with your own household's.

- Make sure your pet can be cared for properly if you fall ill or when you go on holiday.

- Get to know someone else's pets of the same type or breed to find out what the possible problems will be and whether you will be suited to each other.

When you have decided on the type of pet you want and are looking at possible individuals:

- Only acquire your pet from reputable sources, such as:
  - Good recognised and registered breeders
  - Major rescue centres that check potential owners thoroughly
  - Direct from somebody you know well and trust
  - Properly managed pet shops, if you must – but remember that animals will already be under stress by the very fact of being in a pet shop in the first place.

- Check the environment in which it has been kept, to reduce the chance that it is already diseased.

- Check the animal's medical history (including vaccinations and past illnesses).

- Check the history of its parents and brothers and sisters, if possible.

- Choose a healthy animal unless you are prepared for the demands of nursing, the cost of veterinary bills and the possible heartache when it dies prematurely.

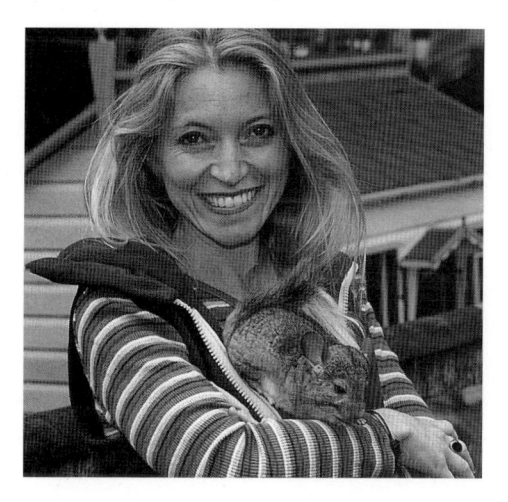

TRUDE MOSTUE + Pets in Practice

- Ask to see the parents if at all possible and ask whether they have been vaccinated
- Ask to see hip dysplasia records in the case of labradors and retrievers.
- Ask whether the bitch and the puppies have been wormed.

Whether it is a pedigree puppy or a mongrel, choose one that is confident and happy. If it approaches you, that is always a good sign. If you are attracted to a puppy that sits in the corner or a little runt hiding under the chair, be aware that its temperament might be less predictable and that runts tend to develop more health problems.

Choosing a cat

There are so many unwanted moggies about that it is only fair to consider one of them, from a rescue centre or from an advertisement in the local papers perhaps, before you decide on buying a pedigree kitten. The drawback to a rescue animal is that its vaccination history is probably unkown and you might be taking trouble home.

With pedigree cats, the variation between breeds is less dramatic than in dogs, but you need to be aware that the oriental breeds, for example, are more dependent on people and that long-haired breeds like the Persian require a lot of coat maintenance. Discuss the problems and the breed's characteristics with the breeders. You can also look at cat magazines for information and for breeders' addresses.

Before you buy, check the vaccination status of the whole litter and the queen and ask to see both parents.

Choosing a reptile

Spend a lot of time finding out all you can, especially about the different reptile species' natural habitat and what you need to offer them to keep them healthy. Find out what part of the world they come from and what conditions they would live in there in the wild. Talk to experienced reptile owners and talk to a reptile shop to make sure that you

---

Trude's helping hand

What to look for in a healthy animal

- Bright shiny eyes
- Alertness and responsiveness
- Healthy shiny coat/feathers/scales and healthy skin
- Sound teeth/beak – overshot or undershot jaw?
- No genetic deformities
- Correct weight and size for its age
- Avoid an animal with dull eyes, dull coat, fleas, a dirty back end or an animal that is thin, pot-bellied or unresponsive.

are reaching the right decision about what type of reptile to buy. Be aware that you need to be able to give space and time to any reptile, and also be aware that there are very strict regulations about importing certain species – make sure your new pet is legitimate.

Choosing a bird

If you want a parrot, you will find it is a lot more demanding than a budgie. Most parrots need as much attention (and space) as a dog. Talk to experienced parrot keepers about different species – your pet shop might be able to put you in touch with the right people. Read as much as you can, especially about the birds in their natural habitat.

No tail to wag

A couple of months ago I met a lovely couple when they asked for their old boxer to be put to sleep. The boxer was about 12 years old, which is a good age for a boxer, but they were devastated and both of them were crying. Then I found out that their other dog had been put to sleep only two weeks before and so they were going through hell. They were very depressed by it all.

After we euthanased their dog the woman came back to see me with her daughter and the daughter's cat. We started to chat about whether the couple would have another dog and we talked about finding another boxer. I asked them to make an appointment to see me so that we could discuss how they should go about it in more detail. The couple made the appointment and we talked about what they should look for in a new puppy. They had been through so much and I really wanted them to get the best dog possible.

They seemed to be set on another boxer and so I talked in general terms as I would to anybody looking for a pedigree puppy. Go to a good breeder and make sure that what you get is what you are looking for. Don't settle for anything less. Go to a breeder who has both the mother and the father so that you can see the temperament on both sides. Talk about the health of previous litters and of the parents to find out if there are any weaknesses in the line.

We also talked quite seriously about finding a boxer with a longer than normal nose. As a veterinary surgeon I like animals that do not look too abnormal; I like dogs that are closer to the wolf rather than dogs with squashed face. Breeds that have physical abnormalities – like the long-bodied and short-legged basset hound and the dachshund, or boxers with a squashed face, or shar-peis with their wrinkled skin – are prone to all sorts of problems and I do not agree with breeding for these abnormal features. We only think that they look good and we do not think about the health issues concerned. I do not believe it is right to breed for abnormalities.

So I said to the couple, 'Whatever you do, go for a boxer with a longer nose.' They both agreed with me and said, yes, they would do that. 'And make sure you get a boxer with a tail,' I said. Their two previous dogs had had docked tails and I feel very strongly against the mutilation of docking. Again, they said that, yes, they would get a boxer with a long tail.

About two months later they turned up with a lovely boxer puppy. I was really pleased to see them and they were beaming with pride. They were so happy with this little dog. His name was George and he had a lovely long nose – a longer nose than was normal for boxers, at least. His temperament was fantastic and of course he was a very happy animal; most boxers are happy by nature and so are most puppies.

But he had a docked tail! 'What's happened here?' I asked them. They told me that they did not have much choice, because the puppy had been docked before they had the chance to tell the breeder that they wanted one with a long tail. They also said to me, with absolutely conviction, 'Actually we think it is best that he has a docked tail because the breeder told us that they get so many injuries to the tail when it is long.'

It amazes me how much people believe the breeders! How can the breeders do this? How can they make such a statement in a serious way when they know perfectly well that it is not true? It is absolutely not true! I see hundreds and hundreds of dogs every single year with long tails, including working dogs, and they have no problems with their tails. I have been in practice for four years and in all that time I have seen only one problem with a tail. I have spoken to many other vets with longer experience and they all agree with me that the breeders' excuse of damaged tails is nonsense. After all, wolves spend a lot of time hunting but they never evolved short tails!

Of course, this lovely couple with the boxer puppy trusted the breeders and believed them. That really hurt – that the breeders could say such a thing, that they abused people's trust in this way. People trust their advice and it makes me really angry that breeders abuse that trust.

So George had a short tail and there was nothing I could do about it. He is wonderful anyway, trying to wag his little stump by moving his bottom from side to side. He has come back for castration because he was becoming a bit frisky, but the docking still infuriates me.

I am sure people are becoming more and more aware about the docking issue. If it had been up to the British public, docking would not exist. It seems to be more a breeder and show-ring fixation. If they want to enter their dogs at the big shows, particularly breeds such as Rottweilers and boxers, they know that the judges will not award prizes to dogs with proper tails. I can understand the breeders' problem in this; of course they feel that they have to dock these dogs if they are after the big prizes. It is all about prestige and money; it is all about showing that their dogs have good pedigrees if the breeders want to make a living from breeding them.

In many ways I feel it is down to the Kennel Club and the judges. They are the people who could quickly make docking unfashionable; and in most cases 'fashion' is all that it is. I realise there are certain working breeds in which it might be beneficial not to have a tail, and I support that, but when it comes to boxers and Rottweilers, Yorkies and cocker spaniels, how many of those breeds are proper working dogs these days? So that argument does not apply to all.

If the Kennel Club were to introduce a rule that docked dogs could not be shown in the ring, the problem would disappear. I cannot understand why such a rule has not been introduced. In some European countries (including Norway) a ban is either imminent or already in place.

The veterinary profession is well aware of the arguments against docking and, in fact, veterinary surgeons are no longer allowed to dock tails; they can be struck off if they do so unless there is a good medical reason for the operation, such as an incurable injury or a sound reason why the dog should be deprived of its tail.

When these regulations first came in, an amazing number of puppies suddenly started coming to the surgery with injured tails, and many vets were forced to dock them. There were nasty rumours about breeders deliberately fracturing tails just to get them docked by a vet.

A client told me recently about a breeder who always docked her own puppies with kitchen scissors. Some vets would rather do the job themselves, with the puppies under anaesthetic, than know that the puppies are being abused in this way by the breeders.

It really makes me angry when people use the injury argument. Why can't they just admit that they think the dogs *look* better with a short tail? It is terrible that we inflict animals with unnecessary pain just because we think they look better without a tail. A tail is an important communication aid and balancing aid for dogs – they communicate through body language – and the tail plays an important role in telling you or other dogs what the dog feels about a given situation. Tail docking robs the dog from communication. I wonder if Rottweilers get into trouble a lot because of misinterpreted body language.

If you choose cosmetic surgery for yourself, that is fair enough; it is your own body on which you are inflicting the pain. But cutting off the tail on a three-day-old puppy is causing them unnecessary pain. I would say it is as much pain as would be inflicted on a newborn baby if you cut off its little finger. How many people would do that?

St Bernard and the fairy

Don't ask me why, but I was once asked to dress up as a fairy and to appear with a St Bernard, waving my magic wand over him. He was a top dog – best of breed, best in show, with a big rosette to prove it. Yet he had entropion (inturned eyelashes, very painful) and really bad hip problems, which were quite typical of his breed. I asked the breeder how this could be and they said these were genetic defects due to inbreeding because so many St Bernards came from a very small gene pool, and they did not want to bring in new genes from countries such as Germany and Poland because that would also bring in bad temperament.

The same has happened with labradors and golden retrievers, many of whom (particularly the retrievers) suffer from hip dysplasia. It seems that when these breeds became suddenly very popular a few years back, they were being bred from, again, a small gene pool and it was possibly this inbreeding that led to joint deformities. In those days any dog with hip dysplasia was usually put to sleep but today we can give them a hip replacement or other surgery, and luckily there are much stricter rules among the breeders about breeding from animals that are prone to the problem. That is how it should be: the (Hip score scheme) onus should be on the breeders to be sensible in their breeding policies.

TRUDE MOSTUE + Pets in Practice

A dachshund on wheels

I met a dachshund on wheels the other day. The poor thing was paralysed, and had been for years, and his owner was asking me about some of his problems. He had a fine old time in his little personal carriage, as it happens: he could still chase balls and chase the cat, though he sometimes got his wheels stuck. But it seems to be accepted among dachshund owners that many of their dogs do become paralysed, entirely because they have been bred for out-of-proportion long sausage bodies and very short legs. If someone asked me for advice on buying a dachshund, I would just say, 'Don't.' Don't buy a breed that has been deliberately deformed and weakened by years of breeding for 'looks'.

Did you know that the fine old English bulldog has been bred in recent years for a skull so wide that a lot of the bitches cannot give birth without having a caesarean? The breeders are actually making the

Two of my good old friends from Warminster. Like dachshunds, these Bassett hounds suffer from being bred with legs too short for their bodies.

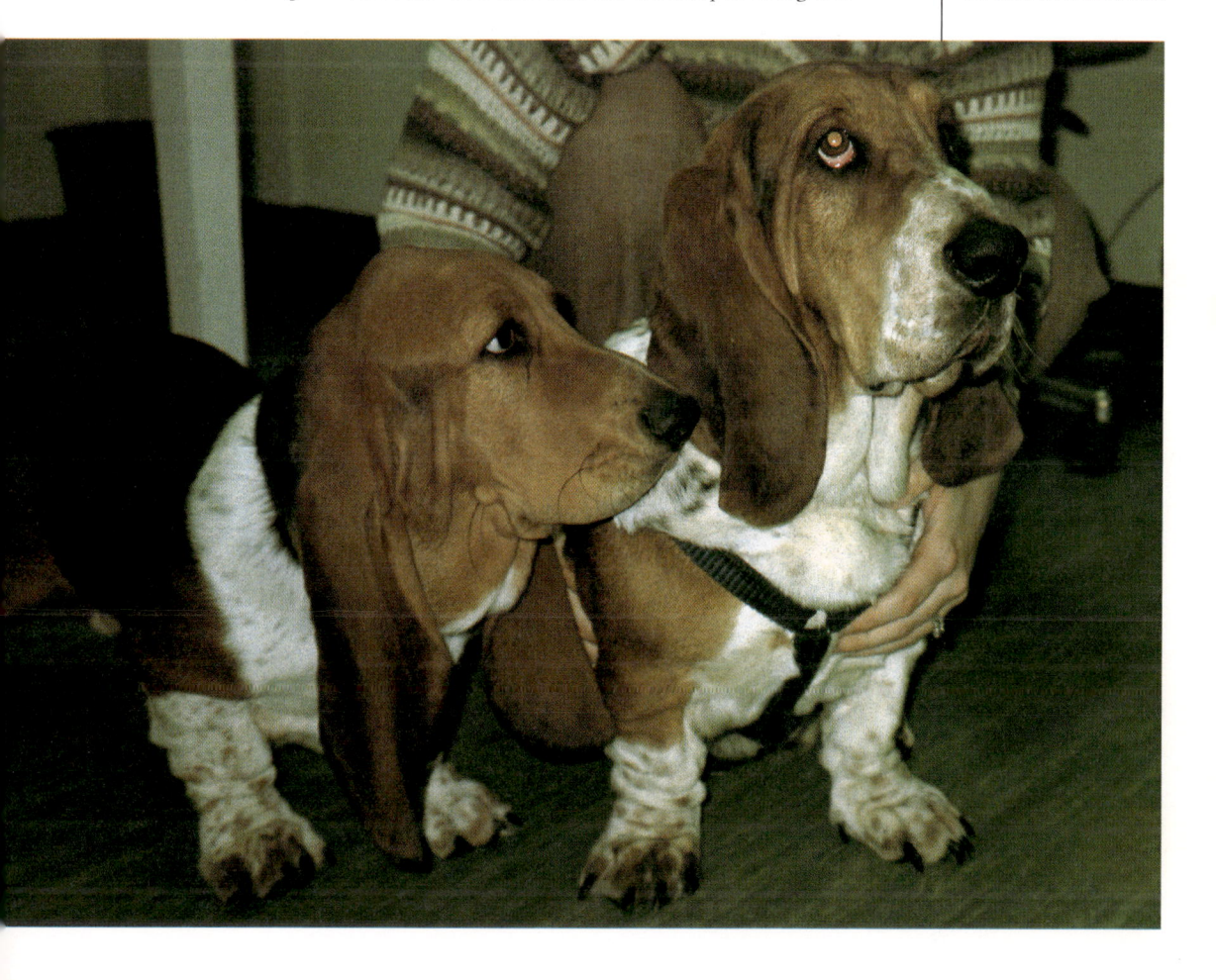

problem worse by deliberately choosing animals with the widest possible skulls. When I was a student we regularly operated on bulldogs in the nose and throat surgery to enlarge their nostrils so that they could actually breathe, and also to shorten the soft palate so that they did not make that terrible noise you sometimes hear in bulldogs and choke on their palate. With some bulldogs, this type of cosmetic surgery has become as routine as giving them vaccinations and worming them, and it is all because that is how the breeders have chosen to develop the breed.

If you look back through the history of domesticated dogs, they originally looked like wolves, yet somehow from that same source we have ended up with the extremes of the chihuahua and the Great Dane. At first, as I have said, breeds were developed for working purposes and for specific jobs, like the German shepherd dog for guarding sheep, the collie for herding sheep, and the labrador for swimming in the sea to help the fishing boats. Why have we bred oddities like the shivering Mexican hairless, and the horribly wrinkled shar-pei that ends up with endless yeast infections in its folded skin? What about all those ridiculously long-bodied breeds, like the basset, whose anatomy almost certainly condemns them to prolapsed discs and other back problems? What about breeds with faces so hairy they cannot see where they are going?

A breeder brought a boxer puppy to see me for his vaccinations and, like George, he had that longer nose just like the old-fashioned boxers and bulldogs that used actually to work. I said to her how good it was to see a boxer with a proper nose, that could breathe and would not snore and snuffle all the time, but she told me she would have to get rid of him (meaning selling him for a low price) because his nose was too long!

Breeders, and people who buy pedigree dogs from them, seem to think that a 'good' pedigree means a healthy dog, but so often it is the exact opposite. I hope this attitude is changing, albeit very slowly, but people still pay for the pedigree and trust that the breeders are the experts, that the breeders know what they are doing. Why do we tolerate these deformed breeds? Surely we should be doing our utmost to get back to dogs that look more like wolves. For years people have been breeding for their own sakes – not for the dogs' good; they have bred something that they think looks pretty or 'different', which is rather like forcing small children to enter beauty contests.

All too often people forget to breed for temperament, and German shepherd dogs are a classic example. So many people choose German shepherds for their good looks without realising that they need very special experienced owners who understand their demanding training needs and know how their dog's mind works. These dogs, more than most, reflect their owners, and all too often you have a nervous owner with a dominant dog that has a nervous temperament. German shepherds have a very strong guarding instinct and are therefore often edgy with strangers; you need to suppress part of that guarding instinct and to build up their self-confidence – but not so much that they are aggressive.

A big advantage of buying a specific breed is that, in theory, you know what the animal will be like when it is no longer just a cute little puppy or kitten. But with dog breeds especially, so many of them have been bred only for looks and not temperament, and so many of them have become a bit nutty, a bit neurotic. Maybe that is why so many people love labradors and golden retrievers, which are usually so easy-going.

Perhaps everybody should pass a test of some kind before they are allowed to have certain breeds of dog! At the very least they need to appreciate that they are taking on a financial responsibility as well as a moral one with any dog – they need to be able to afford the vaccinations and neutering and treatment for accidents, for example. So many people have trouble paying their veterinary bills; they simple do not realise how expensive an animal's treatment can be. Insurance seems to be the way forward these days – it takes away money worries when an accident strikes.

Many people nowadays like to go to a rescue centre and give a good home to an animal, which is highly commendable. But they often also choose a particularly nervous animal, because they feel particularly good if they, and they alone, can win its trust. And, yes, that is a very good feeling, but it is so important that you know just what you are taking on before you give a home to a difficult pet. It is very important that you are prepared to see it all the way through, otherwise you are condemning the animal to going back to a rescue centre time and time again, making its problems worse every time it has to go back. And that is totally unfair on the animal.

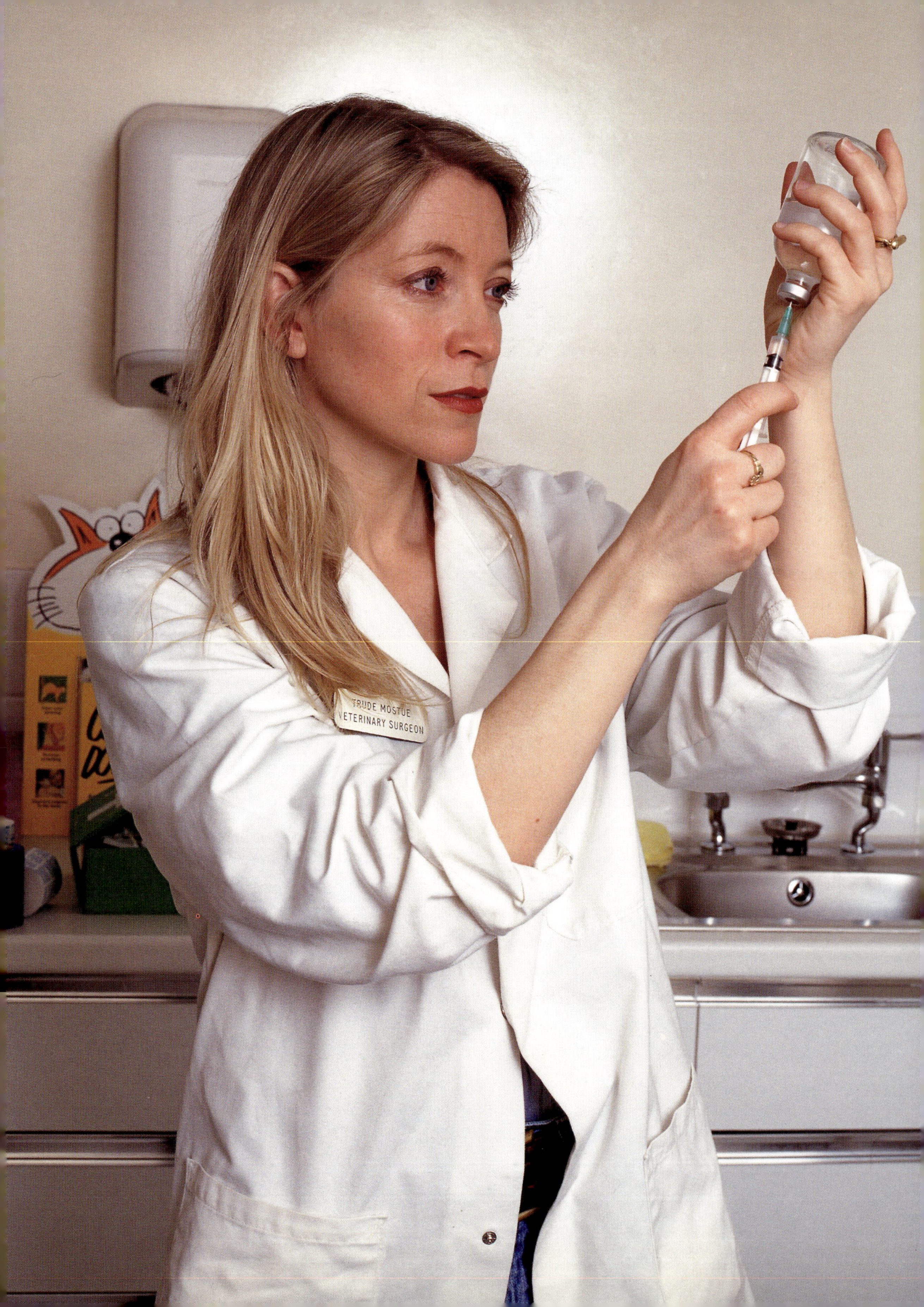
TRUDE MOSTUE
VETERINARY SURGEON

CHAPTER 4
PREVENTION – PROBLEMS THAT CAN BE AVOIDED

People say that an ounce of prevention is worth a pound of cures and most vets would agree strongly with that. Once a problem becomes established, it will take you much longer and cost you much more to fix it than it would have done to prevent it in the first place. In fact, the majority of the conditions and diseases in the animals that come through my surgery doors can be prevented. Helping people to understand how to prevent them is probably one of the most important roles a vet has.

We so often see cases of disease that lead to great distress and even the death of a pet when the whole problem could so easily have been avoided, if only all owners had brought their animal in for vaccinations at the proper times and kept up with booster injections, or if they had taken more trouble to find out about their pet's needs and to keep them fit with the right diet and enough exercise, and an appropriate living area.

Another part of prevention is taking sensible precautions against little biting things like fleas and mites and ticks, before they become too much of a burden for the animal. A lot of my working day is spent in dealing with itchy animals and it can be much more than just uncomfortable for them. For example, mange can make a dog lose large patches of coat, which apart from anything else is very itchy. Severe infestations of some parasites can literally kill a young or weak animal.

I know that sometimes it seems expensive to have all the right jabs given to your pet or to pay for flea products or worming but, believe me, it pays in the long run. It is far more expensive to have to treat an illness than it is to prevent it in the first place; it is far cheaper to control an infestation before it begins to weaken an animal's general health.

The stress of a visit to the vet and an injection pales into insignificance when compared with the stress of a serious disease

By practising prevention, you can avoid such a lot of suffering – both your pet's and, emotionally, your own.

Vaccination

Quite a few potentially fatal diseases can be prevented by the right vaccination routines, not forgetting the regular boosters needed after the initial course. Some of these diseases, by the way, can also affect human beings, so obviously you should do whatever you can to make sure that nobody is exposed to them – including children (your own or someone else's), yourself and other people as well as other animals.

Vaccination is actually the deliberate introduction of a bacterial or viral agent into an animal, which might sound strange but in fact the agent is specially modified (ie. dead or just part of the antigen) so that it does not cause the disease. Instead, it activates the body's immunity to that disease. Each vaccine is for a specific agent or group of agents, but there are also combined vaccines that are given at the same time to protect against several diseases. Vaccines do not necessarily prevent infection completely, but they considerably reduce its severity because the vaccinated animal has a much stronger and quicker response to the particular disease.

To show what I mean, I want to tell you a few stories about pets that had not been vaccinated and what happened to them as a result. I want to make people appreciate how very important vaccination is. The first story is a personal one for me as it is about a lovely little puppy I bought for my mum – a puppy that nearly broke my heart.

Freddie, the present that never was

Just before Christmas and just before my mum's birthday, I decided to get a puppy for my mum and dad. Yes, I know a puppy is not just for Christmas, and it was not like that. My parents had lost their old golden retriever a year earlier and they had been wanting another dog ever since. They just hadn't yet got round to it.

That Christmas I wanted to give them something special and something that would remind them of me in a way, as I was no longer living at home in Norway. I hoped it would be nice to give them a little person, because that is really what a dog is for me. My idea was to find a small male terrier-cross puppy from one of the rescue centres.

I rang lots of places but the only one with a litter of terrier-cross puppies was a rescue centre, on the outskirts of Bath. I went to have a look at the litter and the puppies were gorgeous: they were exactly what I wanted and probably a mixture of Jack Russell or border terrier with something like a collie. It was immediately obvious which puppy I was going to choose – he was a fluffy, beefy little fellow, strong and healthy and very confident, with markings on his face that reminded me of a German shepherd dog. I called him Freddie, after a bus-driver I knew who had a shaggy-dog hairstyle.

There was one possible problem that made me a little nervous about having Freddie. The litter had come from Wales and we have had quite a few puppies and dogs coming over from Wales with parvovirus. There seem to be plenty of stray dogs in Wales that have not been vaccinated and the virus is running through many of them. When I picked up Freddie and took him home I knew that one of the puppies travelling from Wales in the same van as him had had parvo. The puppy had pulled through successfully and as the staff at the rescue centre told me there had been no nose-to-nose contact, I was not too worried.

It was good to get him home. He was a bundle of energy and confidence; he rushed around being a proper little terrier, full of character and killing all the toys I had bought for him. Like any good terrier, size was nothing to him: he would sink his teeth into the sofa and try with great determination to drag it across the room. Everything seemed to be hunky-dory.

Two days later he started to be sick and then he started to have a little diarrhoea. When people get new puppies I always tell them that they should expect some diarrhoea in the beginning, because the puppies are challenged by different bacteria in their new environment. So I kept on telling myself that I should not worry, and everyone at work said, 'You're being silly – don't worry.'

But I had a bad feeling, especially when he started to go off his food and could not keep anything down. On the Sunday evening I decided to take him into work and put him on a drip. From then on he grew worse and worse and I realised that it was probably parvo. Then I learned that another dog from the same litter, which had been taken home by one of the nurses, had gone down with the same thing. There now seemed little doubt that it was parvo.

TRUDE MOSTUE + Pets in Practice

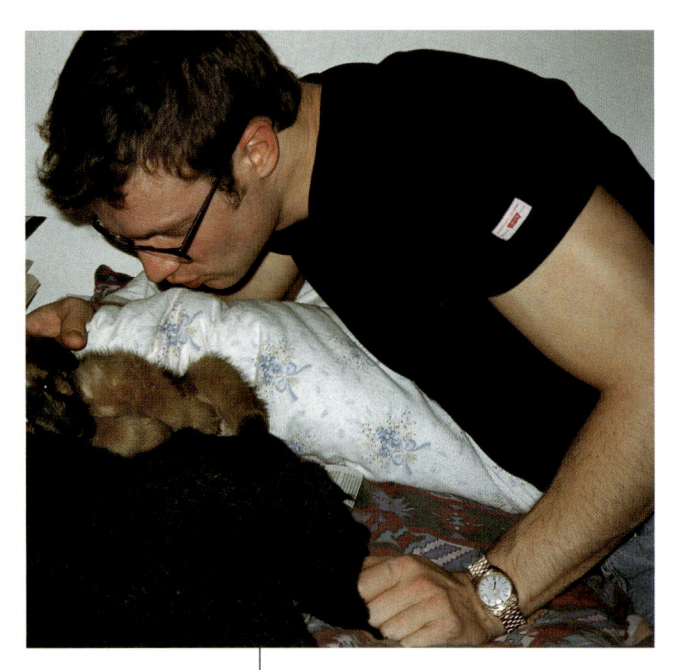

Freddie was feeling very poorly and Brian, my boyfriend, was worried about his condition.

Unfortunately it was too late for me to take any viral tests for analysis, because the results would have been inconclusive. The virus is only shed for the first few days when the symptoms start to show, and at this stage I could not prove from any faecal sample that Freddie did have parvo. Anyway, I thought that he would be able to pull through, because he was a strong little puppy and because I have had cases before and they have been fine. Then again, I had only been in practice for three years so perhaps I was not that experienced.

Wanting to be sure that I was doing everything possible for him, I took blood samples and I took X-rays to make sure that he did not have an intussusception (a distortion of the intestines). Nothing showed up on any of them. By now he had been in hospital about three days and I was still hoping that he would get better.

When I left him that night I was really worried: he seemed to be in so much pain and I gave him extra pain killers to make him more comfortable. I could not bear to see him suffering so much.

When I came in the next morning, I found him dead – still wearing the big bandage on his foot with a drip in.

It was one of the most awful experiences I have had with an animal. I felt utterly helpless; I could not believe that I had failed to pull him through it. It was terrible; I was so depressed, and I could not stop crying. Perhaps it was because I felt that those last days in his very young life were so miserable. Perhaps I should have put him to sleep earlier, but I always thought that we would win through together in the end.

The hard lesson I had to learn was that I could not save everything; that is the reality. It also made me realise that parvovirus is a real risk for all young puppies. Maybe it was a good lesson for me to learn – maybe that is how I should look at it.

Freddie made me feel even more strongly about the importance of vaccination. When owners ask me if it is really necessary to vaccinate their dogs, I usually throw back the question: 'Well, do you think it is necessary to vaccinate your child?' It is because not everyone is vaccinating that we end up with these outbreaks of disease. The aim of vaccination is to eradicate the virus but that will only happen if everyone vaccinates. Freddie's story shows how it can all go wrong: Freddie died for a cause.

By the way, I did manage to get my mum another dog, a pedigree border terrier called Anna, from Oxford. She was successfully sent over to Norway and is very happy there, doing plenty of mousing and ratting. In the end I went to quite a big breeder to avoid taking the same risk; I could not face a similar situation again.

No cure for Tommy

As soon as Mr and Mrs Charlton came in to see me for the first time with their cat, Tommy, Mrs Charlton began to cry.

Now, it is not unusual for people to cry in my office and I realise that people often expect the worst, but it is quite hard for me to know how to take tears. Should I comfort them, should I talk to them, or should I just ignore them? It is not in my nature to ignore something like that and so I asked what was wrong. Mr Charlton was being very sensible and seemed slightly embarrassed about the way in which his wife had opened the consultation, but I thought she was wonderful. She was reacting in a very normal way, because she was so worried about her cat.

The Charltons had had Tommy for 14 years, which is a long time. In the past two weeks she had suddenly lost a lot of weight and did not want to do anything. Not surprisingly, with a cat of that age, Mrs Charlton was prepared for the worst.

I lifted Tommy out of the box. The poor cat was really skinny and and she had that look about her of a typically ill cat. Her black coat was unkempt, her mucous membranes were pale, she seemed badly dehydrated and she was just skin and bones. I could see straight away that there was something seriously wrong with her. We started to talk about different alternatives and I suggested taking blood samples as a first step in diagnosis. They showed that she was positive for feline immuno-deficiency virus (FIV).

FIV is in the same group as the human immuno-deficiency virus, HIV. It works in a similar way, attacking the immune system, and so the animal has a very poor immune response to minor infections that would normally be no problem at all. Another typical symptom of FIV is anaemia: the virus can influence the production of red blood cells and that is what was happening to Tommy.

There is no cure for FIV; all you can do is to support the individual with nursing. Tommy's case was typical of a dilemma in which I often find myself, where I have to make a decision on how far we should go with an animal when I already know that its condition cannot be cured. The Charltons and I talked for a long time about this, which is important because they needed to be aware of the problems and alternatives and of why we were making the decisions that we were making. They needed to know that we were doing everything we could for their cat.

For the time being Tommy was happy at home. She was not as active as she used to be but she was still purring and eating and doing things she always had done, even going out hunting. So we decided to leave her for now and just see how she got on, then, when the day came, we would put her to sleep.

FIV very often comes with the feline leukaemia virus (FeLV) but not in this case. It is transmitted from cat to cat by saliva and cat bites and it can lie dormant in 'carrier' cats for many years. Quite a high proportion of cats are carriers, but it is hard to prove and a carrier cat might never develop any symptoms of the condition throughout its life, which means that it is quite a tricky condition to monitor.

One of the problems facing Tommy's owners was the ethical dilemma of knowing that your cat has FIV and that potentially it can pass the virus to other cats. In such a situation owners need to be aware that it would be irresponsible to let the cat out, in case it meets other cats. With Jodie the problem did not arise: she was so thin by now that she spent all her time indoors.

We continued to give Tommy supportive therapy, which means medication for any secondary infections she might have and rehydrating fluids to drink, but it was very much up to the owner to notice when she was unhappy. I phoned the Charltons every week to see how she was and they would bring her in for a check-up at regular intervals, which gave them the chance to make the decision to put her to sleep when the time was right. Eventually she reached the stage when she was sleeping most of the time and did not even have the energy to walk to her food bowl. When she did walk, she was all shaky, and we felt that the day had come. The Charltons were devastated, of course, but in the end it was all very peaceful. When I finally put Tommy to sleep, she was at home on her favourite sofa, curled up on her owner's lap and purring.

Little Millie

Millie was a little tortoiseshell kitten of about eight weeks old when she first came to see me. She had a ginger brother called Tigger and the owner was slightly worried that Millie was not eating and being as active as Tigger was.

When I examined her she was slightly smaller than Tigger but not dramatically, and she was not really thin; she was eating a bit and I was not too worried. I thought that she was probably more shy than Tigger and it would take time for her to be more confident. There seemed to be nothing abormal: her temperature was normal, her abdomen felt normal and her tests seemed to be normal as well, so I suggested that the owners should give her a little more attention and feed her separately from Tigger, and then come back for the second vaccination in a few days.

A week or so later Millie was brought back to the surgery. Her appearance had changed completely. She had lost a lot of weight and her belly was standing out like a little balloon. She seemed to be happy enough, purring away, but she was very lethargic and her owners told me she was drinking a lot but hardly eating at all. She definitely did not like moving around, because of her big belly. I was very alarmed when I saw this and told the owners that I would check to see what was going on but that, whatever it was, the prognosis would be fairly poor.

Millie was taken into the hospital and I took some samples of the fluid that I found in her abdomen and sent it off for analysis. The laboratory suggested that she might be suffering from feline infectious peritonitis (FIP) virus, which can be seen in very young kittens or cats up to about two years old. You cannot vaccinate against the FIP virus, you cannot cure the disease, nor can you prove definitely that a cat has it. There are no tests available, basically because many cats carry a

TRUDE MOSTUE + Pets in Practice

Cats make great pets. We fall in love with them as kittens and it is tragic if they fall ill. It is essential to take them to the vet if they seem unwell.

similar virus that can give off the same chemical signals as the peritonitis virus but is completely normal for a cat to have in its body. They are both corona viruses and they both give a positive result in tests.

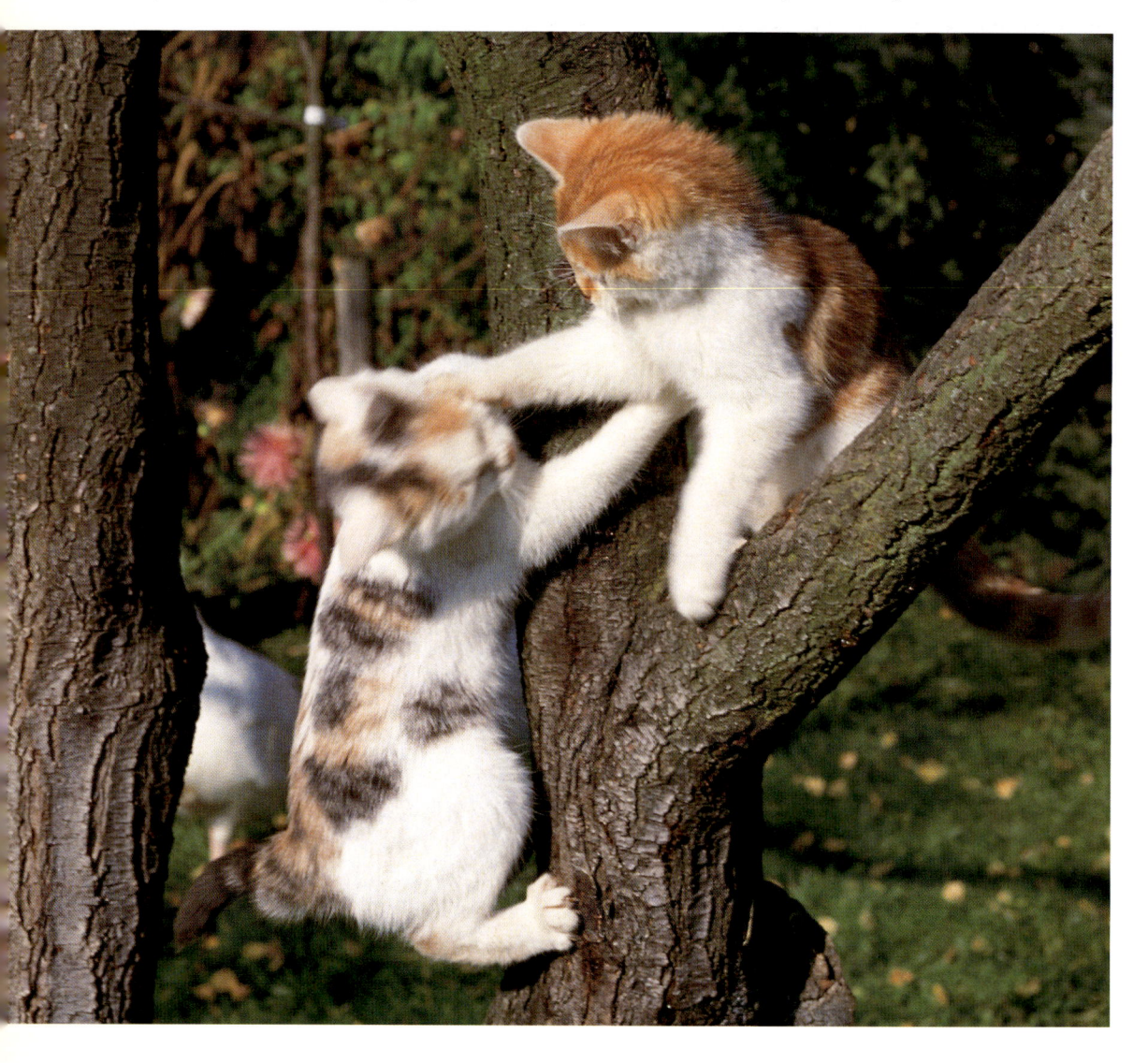

So I could not really prove that Millie had the FIP virus. In the meantime, her condition was becoming much worse and I needed to eliminate other possibilities as quickly as possible. Fluid in the abdomen, for example, can be caused by other things such as tumours but I could not see any tumours on the X-rays. There are also some heart conditions and liver conditions that can cause the same type of symptoms but from auscultation with my stethoscope and from blood tests I could find nothing wrong with those organs. With everything else eliminated, unfortunately it had to be feline infectious peritonitis virus.

As I have said, there is no cure and all we could do was to try to support her and see how she managed. I knew there was only a slim hope for her to survive and we made a decision that if she showed no signs of improvement on supportive medication within 24 hours, we would put her to sleep. And that is what we had to do.

This awful viral condition is transmissible from cat to cat and you might wonder why Millie's brother, Tigger, did not have it too. It all depends on the cat's immune status. Tigger probably had a rather stronger immune system that managed to suppress the virus, while Millie for some reason had a much weaker immune system. She probably caught the virus from her mother: a mother might be carrying it but be strong enough to cope with it herself. Tigger remained healthy, and in due course he came back to be castrated.

Feline infectious peritonitis is frustrating because we still cannot cure it; we can only support the patients and most of them do die, like little Millie.

Vaccinating cats

You can currently vaccinate against feline leukaemia, cat 'flu, calici virus, herpes virus, feline infectious enteritis (feline leucopenia) and chlamydia. The first vaccinations are given at about nine weeks old and you give another injection at 12 weeks old. All of the vaccines need this initial course to bring the level of antibody response to a maximum, so that it is efficient, and they all need yearly boosters. There is a new vaccine on the market that incorporates all these vaccines in one jab, which is wonderful – it means only one jab.

Vaccination against feline leukaemia virus (FeLV) is particularly important if you have a kitten. Strictly speaking, you should take blood samples before you vaccinate against FeLV, to find out if the cat is already positive. To keep the animal's immunity up to date it really needs an annual booster.

Feline leukaemia can be passed to kittens from their mother in the womb or through her milk. It also transmits through saliva, particularly cat bites, which is why it is important for fighting toms to be vaccinated. Feline leukaemia is untreatable and I have seen many cats die from it.

Also, it sometimes works with the FIV virus, creating an immunocompromised animal with anaemia and tumours.

Cat 'flu vaccine can be incorporated into the same injection as feline leukaemia vaccine. You need to be aware that there is more than one strain of cat 'flu virus and not all of them are included in the vaccine. Hence you might see some reaction to some of the strains of cat 'flu virus in cats that have been vaccinated. Cat 'flu may be caused by feline herpesvirus or feline calicivirus.

The chlamydia vaccine is more recent than the other vaccines and it is particularly important if you have a multi-cat household, if you are a breeder or if you just happen to have a lot of cats at home. I do realise that vaccination is expensive when you have a lot of cats but it would cost much more in the long run if one of these viruses should spread through your group of cats. Also, the point of vaccination is to eradicate the condition. If everyone did it, then there would not be a problem and eventually a long way down the line you would not need to vaccinate at all.

Vaccinating dogs

Dogs can be vaccinated against leptospirosis (infectious canine hepatitis) parvovirus, distemper and viral influenza. Thanks to vaccination, distemper is now rare.

With puppies, you usually give the first vaccinations when they are eight weeks old, then repeat the jab at 12 weeks old, though some vaccine makers suggest that the latest jab should be at 10 weeks old. Whether at 10 weeks or 12 weeks, it is most important that puppies do have that follow-up jab when they are older than eight weeks.

Vaccinating other pets

Anyone living in the countryside knows what myxomatosis is. The most common evidence is when you see wild rabbits with puffy, gungy eyes and snuffles. You find them hopping across the road looking very ill and thin and unable to escape quickly; they might appear to be blind and deaf and sometimes seem to sit and wait for predators to grab them.

'Myxy' is an area-related disease; some of my colleagues see many cases but luckily I have seen very few. In the myxomatosis parts of the country you also see the disease in domesticated rabbits, especially if they are out in gardens where there might be wild rabbits coming through at night. The disease is transmitted by fleas and also through grass and rabbit droppings. The domesticated rabbits come into surgery looking anorexic and horrible, with runny eyes and noses.

Rabbits can be vaccinated against myxomatosis and against viral haemorrhagic disease (VHD). In both cases yearly boosters are needed, but if you live in a myxomatosis area it is recommended that your rabbit has a six-monthly booster. Your local vet will be able to tell you whether you are in a high-risk or low-risk area. The vaccination course is started when the rabbit is about six weeks old for myxomatosis and about 10 to 12 weeks old for VHD. You must make sure that VHD and myxomatosis vaccinations are not given at the same time; they need to be two weeks apart.

Ferrets can contract distemper from dogs and should be vaccinated for their own protection. One of the problems with ferrets is that some vets rarely see them and may not always be aware of their particular problems. It is important to use a distemper vaccine that is specifically for ferrets. In fact, some of the dog vaccines can actually cause distemper in a ferret and may kill it.

As with cats and dogs, vaccination starts in the very young animal and then there are annual boosters. Ferrets (and hamsters) can also catch colds and some of the human influenza viruses, so you should try not to handle your ferret too much if you have 'flu.

For most other pets, including small cage mammals (hamsters, gerbils, chinchillas, chipmunks, guinea pigs, mice and rats) and reptiles, there are no vaccines.

Antibodies

You might wonder why vaccination should be started at the ages suggested by your vet. It depends on the level of maternal antibodies that kittens and puppies have absorbed from their mothers. They are born with a certain amount of immunity from the mother, but that natural immunity starts to wane when they reach a certain age – and that's the age when we give them more immunity through vaccines. At about 12 weeks old the maternal antibody levels seem to drop off completely and so it is very important that the young have a jab at that age. But remember that the vaccine will take a week or so to give full immunity and your pet should

TRUDE MOSTUE + **Pets in Practice**

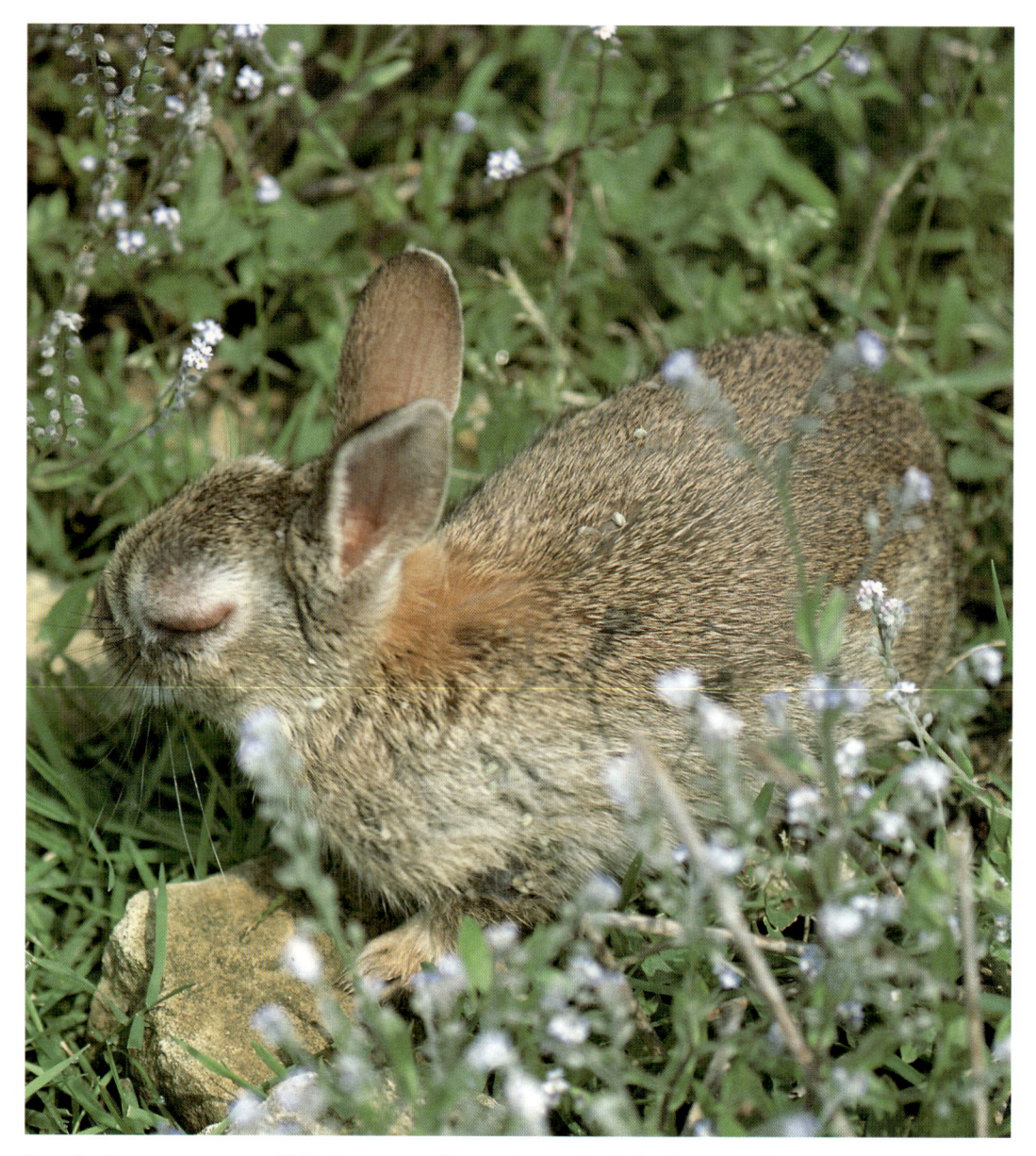

If you live in a myxomatosis area your pet rabbit will need a six-monthly booster injection to avoid looking like this poor thing.

still be kept away from other animals in the meantime.

Initial vaccinations are given when puppies and kittens are younger than 12 weeks, but not too much younger as the existing maternal antibodies would interfere with the vaccine. With puppies or kittens that are more likely to be exposed to certain viruses and certain unvaccinated animals, the first vaccinations are particularly important and can be given a little younger than usual.

Passports for pets

Rabies is a frightening disease and is contagious to nearly all mammals, including humans; it is nearly always fatal in humans. Because of stringent quarantine regulations, Britain has seen only a handful of cases of rabies since the early 1920s, but the British government has recently announced changes in the regulations that will allow some pets to come into the UK without having to go into quarantine. The new scheme is known as PETS, which is short for Pet Travel Scheme.

PETS allows dogs and cats to enter the UK from certain approved countries (mostly European), as long as the animals meet certain conditions. It only applies to pet dogs and cats, so it will not be any good for your pet boa constrictor. The scheme also allows you to travel to and from countries in western Europe with your pet and you need to contact your veterinary surgeon so that they can find out if the country you want to travel in is included in the scheme. Dogs that provide help to the disabled might also be able to travel between the UK and Australia and New Zealand.

The scheme only operates on certain sea, air and rail routes to and from the UK. You need to ask your vet or contact the PETS helpline number for details.

The conditions that pets must meet in order to be allowed to come back into the UK are as follows:
1. Pets must be fitted with a microchip, and the chip must be to ISO specifications (ISO is the International Standards Organization) so that it can be read by a

Trude's helping hand

Vaccines

Different vaccine manufacturers make different recommendations about vaccination regimes and so the timing will vary from practice to practice, but here are some broad guidelines.

Dog vaccines

Against:
- Distemper – Hard pad
- Parvovirus – Diarrhoea and vomit
- Leptospirosis – Liver infection
- Parainfluenza
- Rabies (if your dog has a travel passport)

Give two injections, four weeks apart. The standard regime is at eight weeks and again at 12 weeks old.

Cat vaccines

Against:
- Feline panleucopenia (feline infectious enteritis)
- Cat 'flu (calicivirus and others)
- Feline leukaemia virus (separately or combined with the above two vaccines)
- Chlamydia (in multi-cat households)

Give two injections, the first at nine weeks old for enteritis and cat 'flu and the second at 12 weeks old, with yearly boosters.

Ferret vaccines
- Distemper – a course of two injections, then yearly boosters.

Rabbit vaccines
- Myxomatosis
- Viral haemorrhagic disease

First injection at three months, VHD two weeks later; booster every six (myxo) or 12 (VHD) months.

standard microchip reader; otherwise you have to provide your own microchip reader.

2. Pets must be vaccinated against rabies and given booster vaccinations as recommended. Pets must be at least three months old and they need to have a microchip before they can be vaccinated. The recommendation is for two injections of the rabies vaccine, two to four weeks apart, as the preliminary course and then a yearly booster.

3. Pets need to be blood-tested 30 days after the last injection. If the animal fails the blood test it will have to be vaccinated and blood-tested again. The blood test is only required after the initial vaccination course. Provided that the booster vaccinations are given at the recommended intervals, no further blood-testing will be required.

4. Before travelling, pets also need to have a signed health certificate certifying the rabies vaccination, the microchip and the blood sample. You also need a certificate to show that your pet meets the health requirements for the countries you are visiting or travelling through.

Trude's helping hand

Some diseases you can catch from your pet

- Bird-fancier's lung (pigeons)
- Cat-scratch fever (cats)
- Leptospirosis (rats – causes jaundice)
- Lymphocytic choriomeningitis (mice, hamsters)
- Ornithosis (from various birds, mostly by inhaling dust from their faeces and feathers)
- Pasteurellosis (various small pets)
- Psittacosis (parrots)
- Rabies (mainly dogs, also wild mammals)
- Rat-bite fever (rats and other pets)
- Ringworm (dogs, cats, small cage mammals, birds – by direct contact)
- Roundworms (dogs, cats – Ancylostoma hookworms burrow into human skin; Toxocara cani worms from dog faeces may burrow into eyes)
- Salmonellosis (dogs, cats, birds, reptiles – usually from direct contact with faeces)
- Scabies (sarcoptic mange)
- Tapeworms (various animals – faecal contamination)
- Toxoplasmosis (cats, also other mammals and birds – dangerous for pregnant women in particular)
- Tuberculosis (dogs, cats)
- Yersiniosis (cats, guinea pigs, hamsters)

5. Pets must be treated for certain parasites 24–48 hours before returning to the UK. These parasites include a particular type of tapeworm that can also infect humans, and a particular type of tick. This is in order to minimise the chance of introducing various diseases from other countries. You must have a certificate signed by an official veterinary surgeon confirming that the treatment has been given.

Those are the conditions. Before your pet re-enters the UK the transportation company will check its microchip number and will check the record of rabies vaccination, the blood test results and the certificate of treatment for tapeworm and ticks. It is very important to make sure that you have done all that is required to meet the conditions for the pet and that you have all the paperwork, otherwise your pet might be refused entry or have to go into quarantine when it returns to the UK.

For your own peace of mind when travelling with a pet, ask your local vet about possible preventive treatments to minimise any problems while you are abroad. For example, you could ask for an insecticide that protects against ticks (always a good idea, because ticks do carry some blood-borne diseases).

If you need more information about travelling with pets, you can always ask the Ministry of Agriculture, Fisheries and Food (MAFF) or your local vets.

Parasites

If it wasn't for parasites – blood-drinking things that bite and cause skin problems, things that burrow into an animal's innards and other nasties that feed off their hosts in various ways – quite a few vets would probably go out of business! They say it is a dog-eat-dog world but it is really more like a parasite-eat-dog one. The little beasties seem to be everywhere, and the skin parasites in particular are even happier now that houses are better heated in winter and often offer them nice warm hiding-places and breeding nests like carpets, upholstered furniture and bedding.

Kate the pot-bellied kitten

Kate was a small tabby moggy living in Warminster and she was about six weeks old when she came to see me. She came in with a family of three young sisters: one six-year-old, one of eight and one of 12. They were all very excited about having a new kitten. They had picked up Kate a couple of days before and came in for a check-up, also commenting that her tummy was too big.

When I checked her over she was a sweet little kitten, a typical moggie, purring away and very trusting, but the children were right: she did have an enormous belly. I asked them where the kitten came from. Was it a place where her mother might have been wormed, for instance, and had the kitten been wormed at the vets? I had a feel of her belly. It did seem to be full of something and I was a bit worried it might be worms.

They told me that she had not been wormed and they doubted that the mother had been wormed either, because it was a farm cat. Kate was eating well; in fact as she was eating like a horse. As she was behaving like all other kittens, apart from having a pot belly, I decided to start her off on some wormers. I gave her a dose then and there and asked her owners to come back and see me again the next day.

When they returned they all looked horrified. They told me that Kate had been sick and she'd had diarrhoea and the children said they had found lots of what looked like small pieces of spaghetti in it.

This was because the wormer had started to kill off all the worms inside her and they were coming out in her vomit and faeces. They looked revolting but suddenly her belly was smaller than it had been yesterday. So she had indeed been pot-bellied because of worms.

I talked to the family about worms and how often Kate should be wormed. In general, depending on the wormer, the makers recommend worming kittens every fortnight up to 12 weeks of age. After that, to be absolutely sure, you need to worm them once a month up to six months of age.

For hygienic reasons, especially if there are children in the house, I always recommend worming cats every third month. If cats catch mice and birds, they will have tapeworms; if they have fleas, they will have tapeworms. If they don't have tapeworms they will have a roundworm called Toxocara cati, and that is not a very pleasant little beastie to find on your lap.

It is typical for there to be a heavy worm burden in kittens and puppies that come from homes where the queen or the bitch has not been wormed. The worm larvae can come through the milk, particularly

Trude's helping hand

Worms

The life cycle of the *Toxocara canis* roundworm in dogs:

- The eggs are accidentally eaten by the bitch.
- The eggs become larvae and lie dormant in the bitch.
- When the bitch becomes pregnant, the larvae can infect the puppies in the womb and can also travel into her milk so that the puppies are infected through the milk.
- The larvae can hatch into egg-laying adults inside the puppy until the puppy is 14–16 weeks old.
- Large numbers of eggs can be passed into the environment by puppies and bitches and can infect other puppies and dogs ... and children.

Facts about roundworms

- One adult *Toxocara canis* roundworm can produce 25,000 to 80,000 eggs per day.
- It can grow up to 15 cm in length.
- It can cause toxocariasis in people. In the worst cases, children can become blind.
- The most likely source of contamination is when children are in contact with faeces from dogs.
- The life cycle of the cat roundworm *Toxocara cati* is similar to that of the dog roundworm except that kittens become infected through their mother's milk, not in the womb. There is less risk of infecting humans, because cats bury their faeces.

Facts about tapeworms

- The most common tapeworm spends part of its life cycle in the flea. Flea larvae eat tapeworm eggs. The adult fleas are then eaten by a dog or cat and they release an immature stage of the tapeworm inside the animal, which becomes an adult tapeworm in the animal's gut. Some of these tapeworms can complete their life cycle in only three weeks.
- Some tapeworms pass part of their life cycle in sheep, cattle or rodents. Dogs and cats that hunt might be infected by catching and eating mice and voles.
- One fairly rare tapeworm species (usually found only in Wales and Scotland) can cause disease in humans who accidentally eat the eggs, though the usual host is sheep. Dogs might be infected by eating infected sheep carcases.

Worming

Adult dogs should be wormed at least four times a year, and pregnant bitches more frequently. How often you should worm a puppy depends on the type of wormer but usually every two weeks until it is 16 weeks old.

Adult cats should be wormed every three months. Kittens should be wormed every two weeks up to about 12 weeks old, then once a month until they are six months old.

with bitches. When the bitch gets pregnant her hormones reactivate larvae lying dormant in her muscle tissues, stimulating them to migrate down to the mammary tissue and into the milk so that they can complete their life cycle in the puppy.

My own little puppy, Freddie (the one who died from parvovirus), was full of worms when I first got him. Like Kate, there were worms in his diarrhoea and worms in his sick – it was quite disgusting.

If you have children and puppies in the same household, the most dangerous parasite is the roundworm called Toxocara canis, which can in theory use human beings as an accidental host and can cause blindness in children by burrowing into the eyes. Although it is very rare, most people feel that if there is any chance at all that children might be in danger, however long the odds might be, then it is better to try to prevent it than to wait for that one very rare case.

Worms in other pets

Internal worms are not, of course, the wriggly things you find in garden soil. Instead, they are various types of parasite that spend part or all of their various life-cycle stages inside a host and they are not fussy about whose insides they inhabit. Even a pet grasshopper might be infested with a type of roundworm.

The group called roundworms (also known as nematodes) include flukes and leeches but also all sorts of other parasites in all sorts of living creatures; some of these creatures prefer to live in the stomach, others in the intestines or the liver, heart, lungs, eyes and other organs, and some dig under the skin and into muscle tissue and nerves. In the pet world roundworms don't just attack cats and dogs; they sometimes infest chinchillas, for example, and cage birds. Tortoises and terrapins quite often have them but do not usually show any obvious symptoms until the owner sees something unpleasant in the tortoise's droppings in late summer. Pet snakes are sometimes infested with roundworms and a typical symptom in snakes is diarrhoea.

Tapeworms are even more disgusting and can find their way into most pets and farm animals. They are of several different types and need more than one host to complete their life cycle. One of the most common tapeworms lives in rabbits and hares, while the type that infects cats passes some of its life cycle in the livers of rats and mice. Another type (luckily rare in Britain) starts off in a crustacean, which is then eaten by a fish, which in turn is eaten by a dog, cat or human being. In a human, this particular tapeworm can grow to as much as 60 feet long! (which will keep you slim!) It is not quite so big in dogs but as dogs can pass tapeworms to farm livestock it is very important that farm dogs in particular are regularly wormed. Other tapeworms might infect chinchillas, but more often you find them in hamsters and gerbils, which can pass them to cats. Pet rats and mice sometimes suffer quite badly from both tapeworms and roundworms.

Three little kittens

A couple of years ago a client brought in three tiny kittens from a litter. He was worried because the kittens were lethargic and not moving about much. They were about a week old, and it is quite common for young kittens to die within a week of birth.

When I put them on the table they seemed to be almost lifeless. I checked their gums, which were so pale they were almost white. I wondered what on earth was going on. Then suddenly I noticed fleas crawling all over them. There were fleas everywhere, crawling in their faces, crawling on their bellies, crawling in their eyes – it was awful. I realised that I was dealing with flea anaemia.

It is hard to believe that a little parasite like a flea can cause so much harm but a one-week-old kitten does not have much blood and cannot afford to lose it. If there are a lot of fleas on a kitten, they will literally suck the poor little thing dry of blood.

I took the three kittens straight into the hospital. I was starting to get quite upset, because I felt so strongly that this could have been avoided. We spend a lot of time advising people to treat their cats for fleas, especially when there are young animals about as it can cause them so much more damage than people realise.

The owner was beginning to appreciate the seriousness of the situation and when he understood what had caused it I think he started to feel rather guilty. He agreed to let me treat the kittens. First of all I tried to put a fluid line into one of them but it was difficult: a week-old kitten has not got very big veins. One of the kittens died on the table while I was desperately trying to get the fluid line into the jugular vein of another.

When I did puncture the vein, there was no red blood in the syringe – it was such a pale, pale pink that it was almost white and I could hardly recognise it as blood at all. In fact I kept on puncturing the vein, thinking that I couldn't be into the vein. I have never seen such an anaemic animal in my life.

By now I was getting really upset. One kitten had already died but the other two kept on fighting and we started to take all the fleas off their bodies. We were warming the kittens, we were syringe-feeding them with warm milk and doing everything we could to get them going again.

Then a second kitten died – it was basically too late to save it – but the third one was obviously a real fighter and we did eventually manage to pull him through. We kept him in the hospital for a few days on supportive therapy. The main aim was to get all the fleas off him so that he had a chance to regenerate and recover.

In the meantime the owner went home and sprayed everything with anti-flea preparation, including the queen and the carpets. Quite surprisingly, the queen accepted the surviving kitten when he came home a week later and they were fine, but the owner had learnt a hard lesson.

The reason this case upset me so much was that it was so unnecessary. Most people these days do seem to be more aware that fleas need to be controlled and I always emphasise to clients that it is especially important to protect small kittens from fleas. If they do not, the results can be fatal.

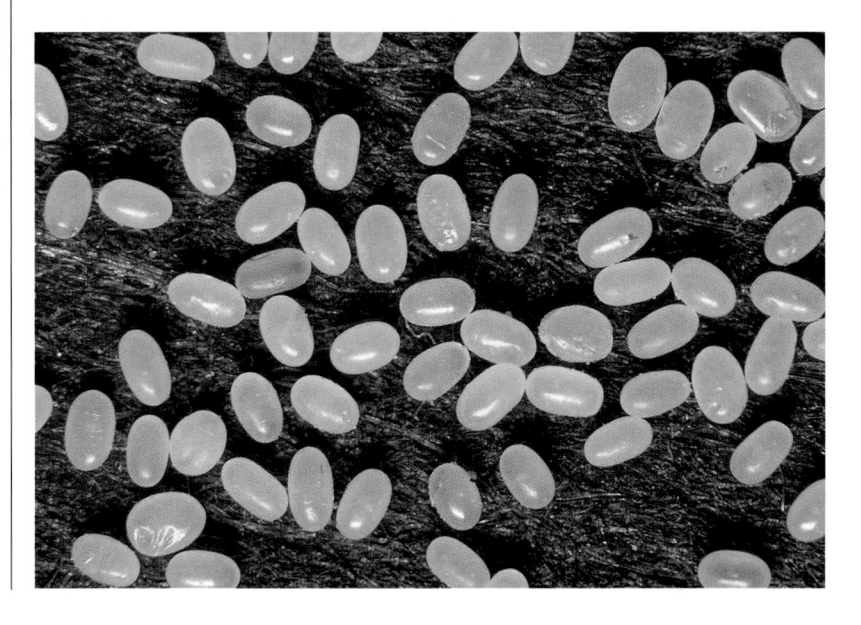

Flea eggs – although fleas are very small they drink a lot of blood. If a kitten has too many of them they can suck the animal dry. Keep an eye out for fleas.

Treating for fleas

The dreaded flea dermatitis, a severe skin infection caused initially by flea bites, is probably the best example of parasite troubles that can be prevented. It might be hard to understand that something as small as a flea can cause such problems and few people take flea infestations seriously at first. Then suddenly they notice that their animal is suffering from flea allergies and skin infection; that is when they do sit up and take notice.

It seems as if a certain level of fleas is deemed to be acceptable, which is perhaps all right as long as you are not dealing with a small animal. If you only knew just how much blood thousands of fleas need to sustain themselves and to lay eggs! When their victim is a tiny kitten, it does not take long for them to drain it of its blood.

Many people are relaxed about fleas and their attitude is that animals will always have them. But there are so many good anti-flea products on the market now that you, too, can have a flea-free animal if you use them on a regular basis.

Fleas are not just uncomfortable for your pet. They can also transmit diseases and can cause chronic allergic reactions. They can carry one of the stages of tapeworms, too, so if your cat has fleas you should always worm for tapeworm as well.

Fleas tend to be seasonal – or they used to be. I find that there are big flare-ups in the springtime and autumn, when for some reason people are less diligent with their flea treatment or when they start to switch on the central heating. Once we get a cold spell we always have people coming into the surgery and saying with surprise that they have loads of fleas around and asking what they can do about their flea-ridden animals.

If you have central heating you should, in my view, use flea preparations all the year round, because the fleas will be around all the time – they no longer lie dormant for very long. Not only should you treat the animal; it is equally important to treat the carpets, because although the fleas will lay their eggs actually on the animal, the eggs drop into the carpet and it is deep in the carpet that the larvae will develop. Not a nice thought is it?!

The choice of flea preparations used to be only sprays and powders but now there are also 'spot-ons'. These are small vials that contain a drug and you just open the vial and squirt it directly on to the skin of the animal: between the shoulder blades for a dog, but at the back of the head for a cat, because cats are so flexible that they can turn round and lick it off from between their shoulder blades.

Although spot-ons are a little more expensive than sprays and powders, they are good and they are easy to apply, which means that people are more likely to use them regularly. This is particularly the case with cats, which hate being sprayed anyway. Spot-ons are also less hard work to apply to medium-sized and bigger dogs.

One of the latest flea preparations is really a contraceptive for fleas – it makes them infertile. It is a good product but it does not actually kill the existing fleas; it just stops them from breeding. It comes as an injection to be given once every six months (you inject the pet, not the flea!), or as an oil preparation to be put in the food once a month.

If you are dealing with a lot of fleas I recommend using sprays for the carpet and using spot-ons or sprays for the animal, depending on what sort of animal you have and how easy they are to handle. If you have asthmatics in the house or small children crawling about on the carpet and you are worried about the residues left from an insecticidal spray, then you might prefer to use the contraceptive preparation.

Looking for flea dirt at home

Very often people say to me, 'My animals don't have fleas, I haven't seen any.' The trouble is that fleas run so fast and jump so fast that you very rarely see them on the animal.

The best way to find out if your animal has fleas is to search for flea dirt rather than the fleas themselves. Brush through the animal's coat and put the brushings from the comb on a wet piece of white tissue paper. The tissue paper will slowly turn red if there is flea dirt there. If you do see live fleas running around, then you have a major problem.

Itchy cats

Cats with fleas can be really tricky because they like to groom. They will clean themselves so well that they clean away all the evidence of fleas. Some come into the surgery with big scabs on their backs and loss of hair along the back and on the flanks. This is usually because they have been overgrooming themselves. Instead of scratching at the itchiness as a dog would, with their claws, cats prefer to lick their coats and so they

Trude's helping hand

Fleas

- There are several types of flea preparation, including sprays, powders, spot-ons, injections, oral products and shampoos. Use the one best suited to the animal and the level of infestation, and the one that you find easiest to apply.

- Use the flea preparation regularly, and use it throughout the year if your home has central heating.

- Treat the animal to get rid of adult fleas, and treat the environment to destroy eggs and larvae. Flea eggs drop deep into carpets and bedding, and the larvae develop there.

- To see if your animal has fleas, brush its coat and put the brushings on to a wet piece of white tissue paper. The tissue paper will slowly turn red if there is flea dirt.

Facts about fleas

- An adult flea can live for about 10 to 20 days.
- One female flea lays 20 eggs a day.
- Eggs, larvae and pupae can stay in the house for more than a year before becoming adult fleas.

- Fleas are not host-specific. Cats, dogs, rabbits and ferrets can get fleas. Fleas may bite humans too.
- Pets can pick up fleas by being in contact with other flea-infested animals.

Flea life cycle

- A small brown egg is laid in the environment and hatches into a larva.
- The larva remains in the environment and feeds on flea droppings and organic debris.
- The larva becomes a pupa.
- The pupa waits anything from two weeks to 18 months until conditions are just right for hatching into an adult.
- The adult flea lives on its host; its life span is 10-20 days.
- The adult female lays eggs on the host; the eggs drop off host and into the environment to hatch.

Most of the flea's life cycle is spent off the host, i.e. in the environment. The life cycle is from three weeks to two years.

---

are constantly dragging the hairs with their very rough tongues, causing traumatic injury to the hair strands.

In any allergic animal that is itchy, the most common cause is fleas and so my first task to is find out whether the animal is already being treated for fleas. Even if there is no obvious trace of fleas or flea dirt, the animal needs to be treated first for fleas, to exclude this possible cause of the itching. If a vet is enthusiastic and really wants to prove it, samples of the cat's faeces can be sent off for analysis and you might

TRUDE MOSTUE + **Pets in Practice**

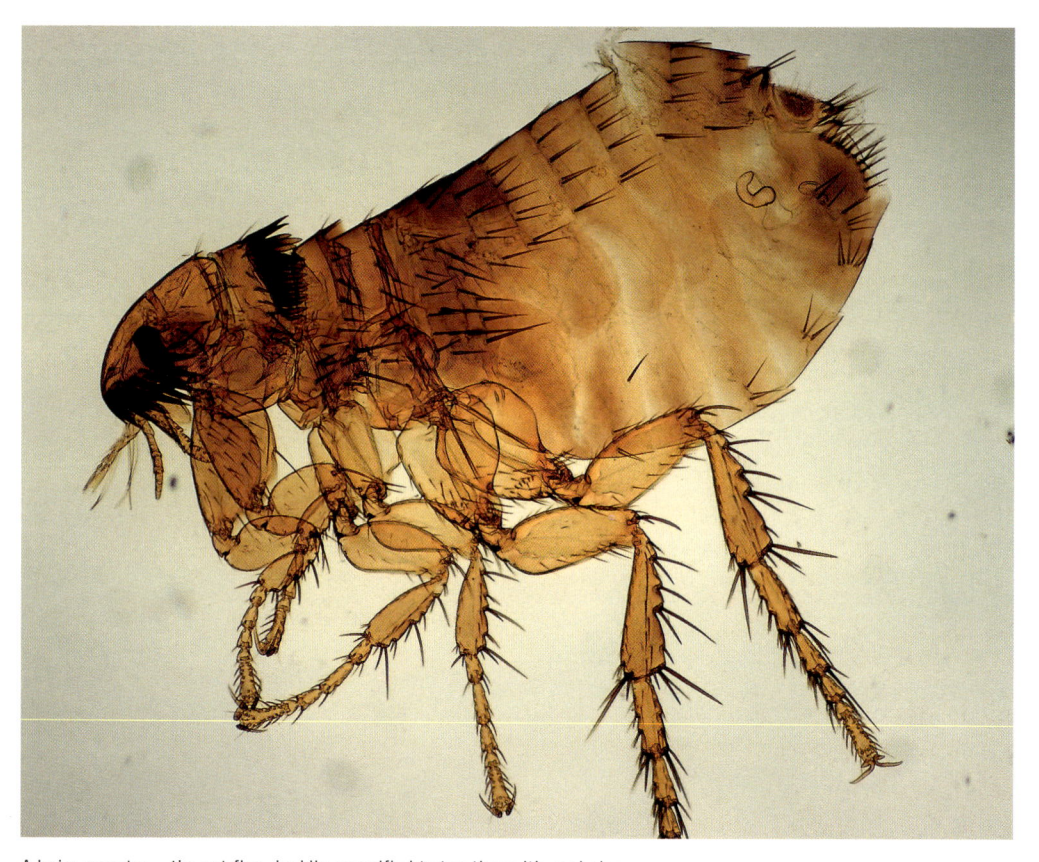

A hairy monster – the cat flea, luckily magnified to ten times it's real size.

Trude's helping hand

Mange mites

- Sacroptic mange mites (fox mange) have round bodies and eight legs. Males have suckers on all but the third pair of legs; females have them on the first two pairs only.

- The egg hatches either in female's body or after being passed by her.

- After two to four days, the egg is a six-legged larva. The larva burrows its way out of the skin.

- After another two or three days, the larva becomes an eight-legged nymph.

- After another three or four days, the nymph becomes an adult and fertilisation takes place.

- In two to four days the female adult starts to lay her own eggs in the host's skin.

The whole cycle from egg to adult could take as little as seven to 11 days. The life cycle lasts for three to four weeks. New batches of eggs are laid every 10 to 14 days. Hence why you have to treat twice and sometimes thrice at two-week intervals.

find fleas in the poo, but not many people go that far!

Itchy rabbits and ferrets

Rabbits can get fleas, too. With rabbits, fleas are not such a big problem as in dogs and cats because rabbits do not live in carpeted rooms, but remember that rabbit fleas can carry myxomatosis and VHD disease from wild rabbits.

Rabbit fleas look quite similar to those you find in dogs and cats. Have a look through your rabbit's coat and keep an eye on it, and anyway keep your rabbit up to date with vaccines against these two diseases. You need to consult your veterinary surgeon about suitable flea products for rabbits because most products are not licensed for use in them and the animals may react to them.

Ferrets can also get fleas, especially cat fleas. Ferret problems are often similar to those of cats and you can treat ferrets with the same flea products as for dogs and cats, but bear in mind that their is no license to use these preparations in ferrets. Discuss the preparations with your vet.

The mighty mite

Fleas are not the only little parasites that can make your pet itch so badly that it loses somes of its coat. An even nastier creature is a burrowing mite called Sarcoptes scabiei that causes sarcoptic mange in dogs. There is only one species of this mite but several different varieties affecting animals such as horses, cattle, sheep, pigs, dogs and foxes. The mite lives on its host for all the stages of its life cycle but can live in the environment and be passed from one animal to another by

---

Trude's helping hand

Tick life cycle

- The egg is laid in the ground and hatches there into a larva.

- The larva climbs up on to Host 1 (a passing mammal) and feeds on the host's blood. When it is full, the larva drops off and falls to the ground.

- The engorged larva on the ground moults and becomes a nymph.

- The nymph climbs up on to Host 2 (another mammal, of the same or a different species) and feeds on the host's blood. When it is full, the nymph drops off and falls to the ground.

- The engorged nymph moults and becomes an adult.

- The adult climbs up on to Host 3 (again, any mammal will do), feeds on the host's blood and mates. When a female adult is full, she drops off and falls to the ground to lay her eggs.

The whole cycle takes anything from two months to two years.

Ticks are not host-specific.

TRUDE MOSTUE + Pets in Practice

Trude's helping hand

Prevention: regular health checks for your pet

Dogs

- Daily: grooming and checking for parasites. Watch out for wet eczema.

- Weekly: floppy-eared dogs (e.g. spaniels) – check for redness, soreness or itchiness. If there seems to be a *lot* of earwax, clean with special ear-cleaners from your vet or pet shop, but it is normal for all dogs to have *some* earwax all the time.

- Monthly: check claws to see if they need trimming, especially dew claws; check for worming.

- Yearly: have an annual check-up at the vet for vaccines and for basic systems (heart, chest, abdomen etc), especially with older animals; also weigh to see if losing or gaining weight.

Cats

- Weekly: grooming for long-haired breeds; check ears of cats that hunt out in the fields.

- Monthly: check claws for trimming (indoor cats – outdoor cats usually keep their own claws trimmed); ask vet for advice about suitable claw-clippers for cats; check for worming if cat is a hunter.

- Yearly: vaccine boosters; weight check; worming supplies.

Rabbits

- Daily: check for mucky back-end in summer in case of maggots; check for other parasites (e.g. 'walking dandruff' mites); check that the rabbit is eating properly.

- Weekly: clean out the hutch etc.; check growth of teeth.

- Every six months: booster vaccination for myxomatosis.

- Yearly: booster vaccination for VHD.

Small furries

- Daily: check that there is clean drinking water.

- Weekly: cleaning routines; check for parasites.

close contact. It is sometimes spread to dogs from wild foxes and is not usually host-specific.

Rabbits tend to get other sorts of mites in their ears and in or on their skin, which is very uncomfy for them indeed. The mites can make tufts of their hair fall out from very sore red skin. Ferrets often get the same sort of mites as cats and dogs but one sort can lead to what ferret keepers call foot rot. The problem is that similar foot symptoms can be caused by distemper and so a vet needs to be sure of the cause.

Gerbils sometimes come in with mites, and again this is often made worse by a poor diet. Guinea pigs and hamsters quite often get various mange mites that make them itch like mad; both hamsters and rats go quite bald when they have lots of mites, which is usually because of bad husbandry or stress. When an animal is bored and lonely, it does become stressed and the mites are quick to take advantage of its lowered resistance.

Occasionally guinea pigs may get lice. Like chinchillas, guinea pigs sometimes chew their own or their companions' fur and sometimes this habit becomes so bad that almost all the hair can be lost. It is a habit that can be quite difficult to break.

Some cage birds suffer from mites. Canaries seem to be more vulnerable to lice (which don't seem to like budgies); ticks are sometimes found on larger cage birds, and the sort of red mite found on chickens might transfer itself to canaries, pigeons and larger cage birds. Red mites lay their eggs in cages and nestboxes rather than on the birds so the whole cage will need a thorough treatment as well as the bird.

Other skinny problems

Snakes get mites, too, and so do lizards (including chameleons, geckos, skinks and iguanas as well as the native slow-worm). They also suffer quite often from ticks. These parasites can really weaken a reptile that is already in less than the best of health and vivarium will need a good clean-out and disinfecting before you can be sure it is clear0. Vets often see snakes with ulcerated 'scale rot' or with blisters, both caused by damp and dirty living conditions, but the main skin problem with reptiles is being unable to slough off the old skin, usually because the environment is too dry.

Ringworm is another nasty – it is caused by various parasitic fungi that live on the skin or hairs of animals, including dogs, cats (which sometimes catch it from mice), rabbits, rats and pet mice occasionally, chinchillas, gerbils, guinea pigs and hamsters (quite common in both), hedgehogs, poultry, cattle, horses and people. The most obvious signs that these fungi are present are round skin lesions, usually raised and crusty and not always itchy, and the hair in the patches falls out. Ringworm can be highly infectious and some people do not realise that, for example, a child can catch ringworm from a cat or guinea pig.

I quite often see skin or fur problems with small cage mammals and usually these are caused by inappropriate diets or wrong handling. For example, if you handle a little chinchilla too roughly it will shed patches of its fur, leaving clean bare skin. Chinchillas also get this 'fur slip' during fights. Another problem I sometimes see is fur chewing, when a chinchilla chews either its own or its mate's fur, and this is usually because of boredom or a wrong diet.

The case of the exploding tumour

There was an emergency phone call one day, when I was on call. Apparently a tumour on a cat's head had 'exploded' and there was blood everywhere. Off I rushed, but when I inspected the cat I found that the 'tumour' was a tick that had been feasting on the cat and was full of its blood. The cat had scratched at the tick and hence all the blood.

This was by no means the first time a tick had been mistaken for a tumour – in fact it happens a lot! Indeed, most people seem to think ticks are tumours when they see them for the first time. They are disgusting to look at but rather interesting parasites.

The tick is actually a tiny little creature, with biting mouthparts that will attach to the skin and suck blood, and it has an expandable little body that swells into a greyish balloon when it has gorged itself on blood. Unless you are looking for ticks, you will not notice them when they first attach to the skin because they are so small, but they very quickly fill up with blood and then they look like little grapes. The typical story is when people are sitting peacefully at home in the evening, grooming their dog or cat, and suddenly they find this big 'tumour' on the pet's head.

The trickiest part of dealing with ticks is to remove them properly without leaving the biting parts still embedded in your pet. I often hear of people trying to kill ticks with things like nail varnish remover but what happens is they kill the tick while it is in the skin and leave it to dry out; then when they try to remove it the head part remains buried in the skin and festers there. This can be the focus for the formation of a little abscess later. Rather than trying to kill the tick while it is still latched in place, what you really want to do is persuade it to drop off all in one piece, which it usually does anyway once it has had its fill of blood. Then it falls on your carpet and leaves a stain!

There are plenty of good products on the market that can prevent tick infection and so ticks need not be a problem. In fact, in general they seem to be more a problem for the owners than for their pets.

Most owners now seem to groom their pets and keep a good eye on them, which greatly reduces the chance of heavy tick infestations.

Types of ticks

Ticks seem to be seasonal in certain parts of the country and there are several different species. In Britain you are most likely to find the castor-bean tick, the British dog tick and the hedgehog tick, and all of them can happily jump on to another species of mammal, including your pet and yourself. Other types of tick are more common in different parts of the world and might be a problem if you take your pet abroad.

The castor-bean or sheep tick is common in rough grassland and moorland. It seems to have two peak periods of activity: one between March and June and another between August and November. It is often found on dogs that live or walk in the countryside and so those periods are when you should be most alert and have a good search through your dog's coat every day, especially if the coat is very heavy and the dog has been out on the moors a lot. The tick hangs around in the grass and jumps on to whatever animal happens to be passing when it is hungry.

Believe it or not, when this tick sucks blood it increases its bodyweight by 200 times. The reason why castor-bean ticks are quite dangerous in Britain is that they can cause anaemia in their victim if enough of them are feeding on it. Also the lesions they can cause in sheep attract blowfly strike and, more seriously, these ticks can transmit the Babesia organism to livestock (which causes red-water disease in cattle and sheep) and tick-borne fever and louping-ill. They can also transmit Lyme's disease to cats.

The so-called British dog tick seems to be mostly a problem in kennels and other buildings, where the tick will survive in small cracks in the floors and walls. If there are a lot of ticks, they will cause a lot of itching and will require a lot of food – which, of course, is blood, and so the dog becomes anaemic. Dogs also usually lose some hair.

Despite its name the hedgehog tick will move on to dogs and ferrets as well as hedgehogs, and it causes the same sort of problems as the British dog tick. It is quite commonly found on suburban dogs and cats in Britain. Like other ticks, it can live in the environment just waiting for a passing host.

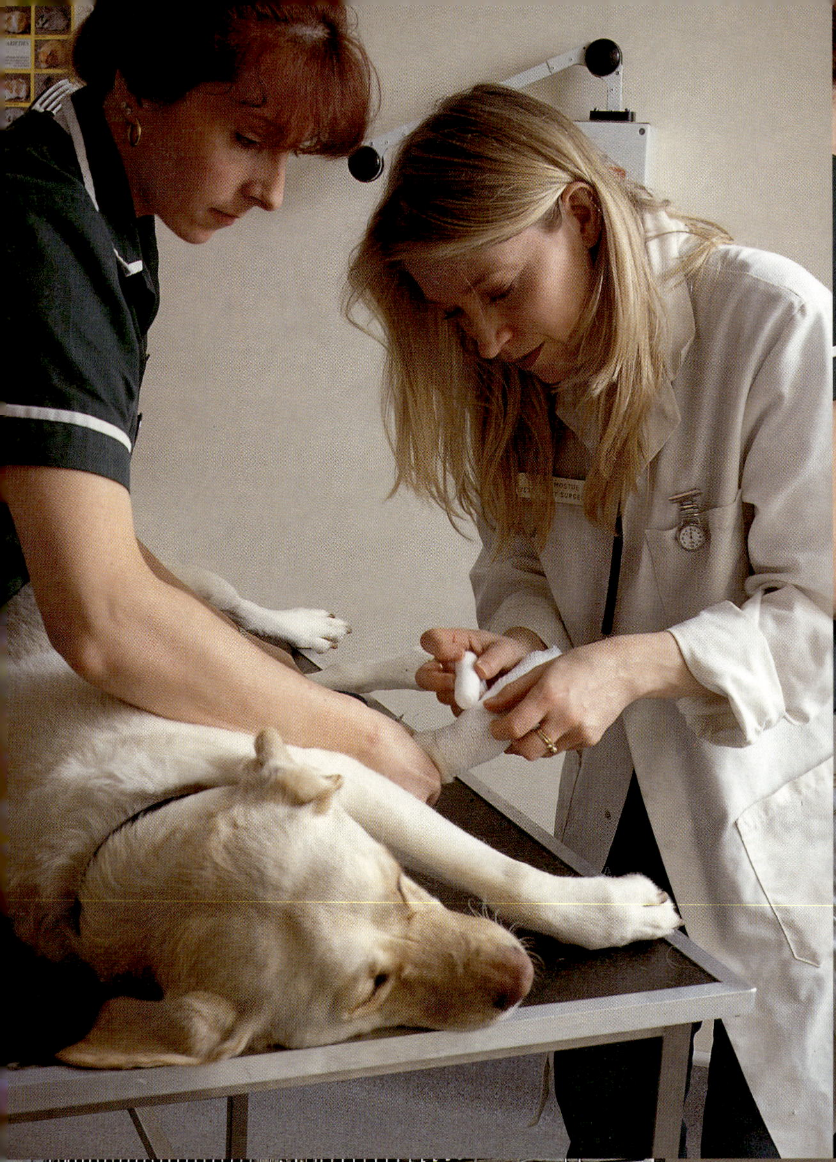
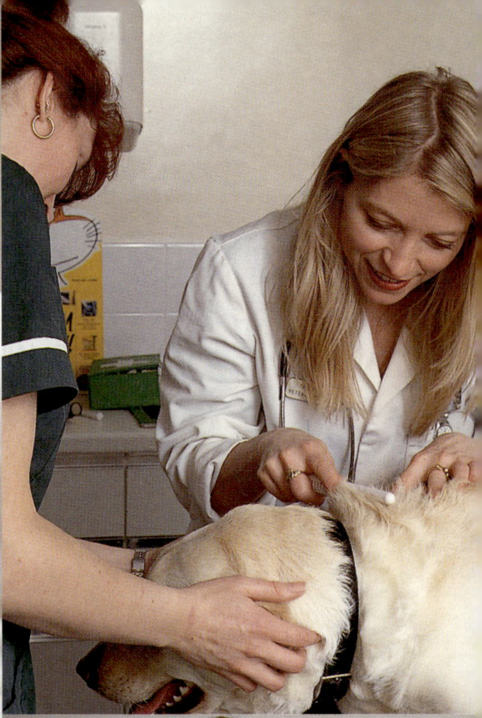
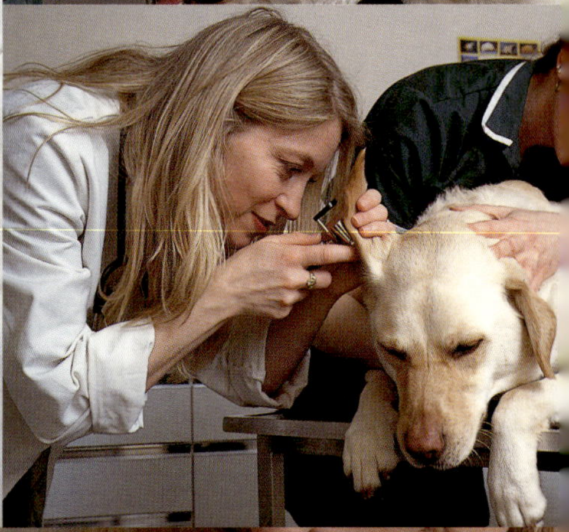
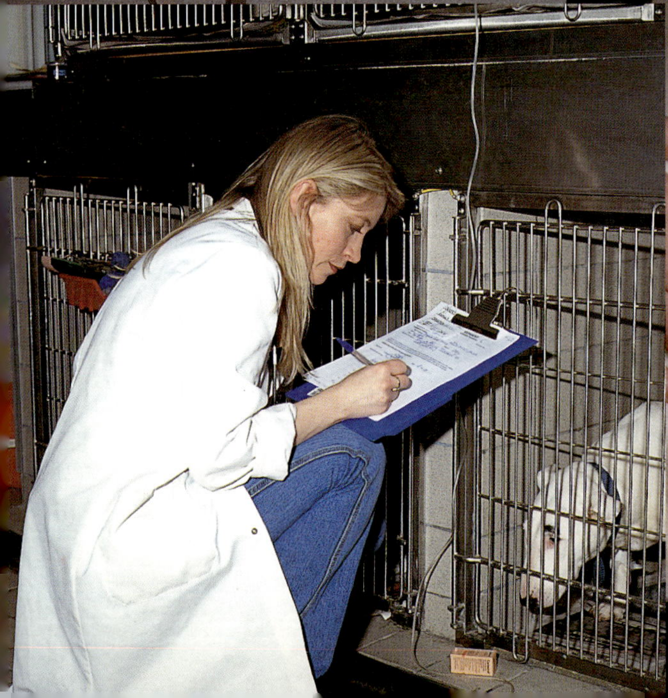
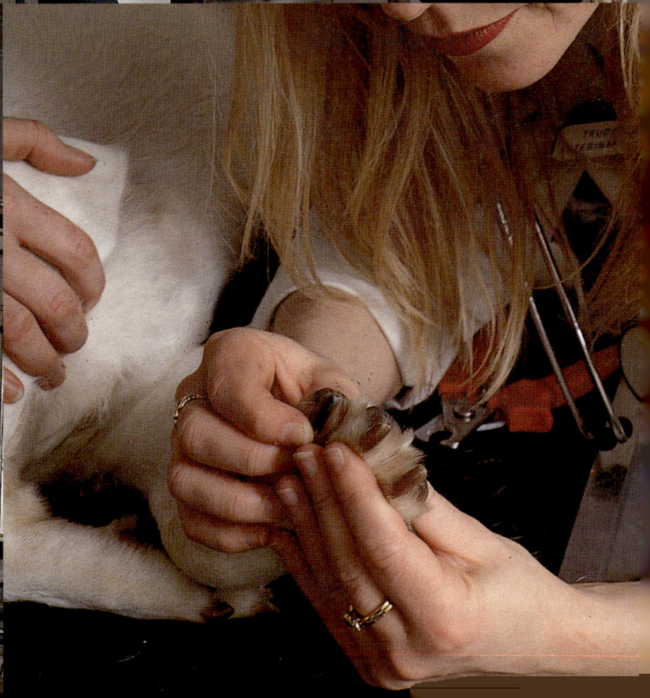

CHAPTER 5

KEEPING FIT

Apart from the excitement of emergencies and births, and the challenges of behavioural problems, most of my work in the surgery is with pets coming in for routine vaccinations and treatment for parasites, or for everyday matters such as overgrown teeth and claws, obesity, lumps and bumps and just generally growing old.

Teeth

Teeth problems are very common, particularly in dogs, cats and rabbits and of course chinchillas. Poor teeth, rotten teeth and a build-up of tartar are some of the most common causes of pain in pets, especially cats. Not only is there pain and discomfort but teeth problems can also cause septicaemia. Bacteria from the mouth can enter the bloodstream and affect the kidneys and the liver, creating more serious difficulties.

One of the problems for dogs and cats is that they tend to be given a lot of tinned food these days – food that does not 'challenge' the teeth. In the wild, of course, they would not get their food from a tin or from sitting by the fridge; they would eat small animals complete with the skin and bones, which would keep their teeth well polished and in prime condition. I have worked with the lions at Longleat and lions in Africa and the latter have amazingly clean, white and beautiful teeth, even when the animals are really old. I could see at close quarters how efficient skin and bones are for keeping the teeth in good condition (luckily, the lions were tranquillised at the time!)

All of the cats and dogs that come in to see us have their teeth checked, and every day we do several 'dentals'. By that I mean mainly

Regular routine check ups at the vets will keep your pet healthy and happy.

113

descaling and polishing the teeth and sometimes tooth extractions. It is sad that we need to do so much of it but very few of the animals seem to have good teeth, basically because they are eating soft food. Feeding dry foods helps, and biscuits, but they still do not offer the teeth the same resistance as would the food the animals might eat in the wild.

The smaller dog breeds tend to have worse teeth problems than the larger breeds. I do not know why but I suspect that little poodles, for instance, and little King Charles spaniels are given more soft foods. Perhaps people spoil them more.

There is no excuse for bad teeth in dogs and a lot of research has looked at how to improve dental hygiene in pets. For example, there are now dental chews that dogs and puppies can be encouraged to chew; there are gels that can be put on the teeth to help to prevent a build-up of tartar; and, if you are brave, you can brush your dog's teeth regularly. There is plenty that you can do to keep your dog's teeth healthy.

Special dental chews and gels are also available for cats and the latest idea is to 'weave' special fibres into biscuits so that they are more 'chewy' and help to clean the teeth that way. These biscuits are already available for dogs and soon will be for cats as well which, for the cat, will be a lot more like chewing on a nice mouse!

People seem to assume that as long as the animal is eating, it is fine, but that is wrong. It is most important that you check your pet's mouth regularly, however well it is eating. These checks will incidentally help the vet by getting the animal used to having its mouth handled, and you should start when it is still a puppy or kitten.

In general, vets now recommend a weekly teeth hygiene routine of some kind. As well as offering some of the chews that are on the market, you can brush your animal's teeth if it will let you. To get it used to the idea, start by using just your finger to rub your pet's teeth and gums as if your finger were a brush, then after a few days put some special dog or cat toothpaste on the finger (don't use your

Trude's helping hand

Dogs and cats need clean teeth

- Dogs and cats eat too much soft food.
- Dog food and biscuits are better for both dogs and cats.
- Dental chews are available from pet shops and vets.
- Special cat and dog toothpaste is available from pet shops and vets.
- Gingivitis and build-up of tartar on a dog's or cat's teeth can cause not only discomfort and pain but also systemic disease such as liver and kidney problems.

own toothpaste) and clean the teeth that way. In due course you can use a suitable brush, which means you will be able to clean the inside of the teeth properly as well as the outside. It is important to be gentle when you brush your pets teeth as they have very tender gums.

Fred Manley's tusks

It was a rainy morning in Warminster when I met a gorgeous rabbit called Fred at a branch surgery of the Garston veterinary group. He was a French Lop – big, fluffy and grey, with fat cheeks – and I was totally charmed by him straight away. Unlike many rabbits, he was so easy-going that he even let me look in his mouth without any fuss.

He had come in because of chronic problems with his teeth but his eyes were also bad, discharging and sore. He was typical of a lot of rabbits in that he had a maloccluded undershot jaw, which meant that his lower incisors grew almost straight into his nostrils. Malocclusion in rabbits is due to several factors, two of the most important ones being cross-breeding and unbalanced diet.

Rabbits' teeth are open-rooted and grow continuously – they can grow at a rate of two centimetres a month unless they are worn down by chewing on sticks or by grinding together. Most rabbits with Fred's problem need to have their incisors trimmed as often as every three weeks. In the wild, of course, they would die, but because they are kept as pets and we are soft-hearted, we help to keep them alive.

Fred's teeth had been cut many times. One of them had just broken off, because it was so brittle, and there was only a little stub left in his gum. His upper incisors curved backwards, almost puncturing the hard palate. From his lower jaw, pus oozed from the edges of the base of the teeth. His gums felt very hot to the touch and he flinched when I touched the sore teeth. The skin around his eyes was red and sore from the discharge.

Although he was by nature a very tough rabbit, all of this was too much for him. His owner, Mrs Manley, told me that he still enjoyed jumping around in the garden and eating all the garden plants but I quickly realised that she was getting fed up with bringing him down to have his teeth clipped so often. I suggested the possibility of extracting the troublesome incisors, which she thought might be a good idea but she was worried about the anaesthetic.

TRUDE MOSTUE **+ Pets in Practice**

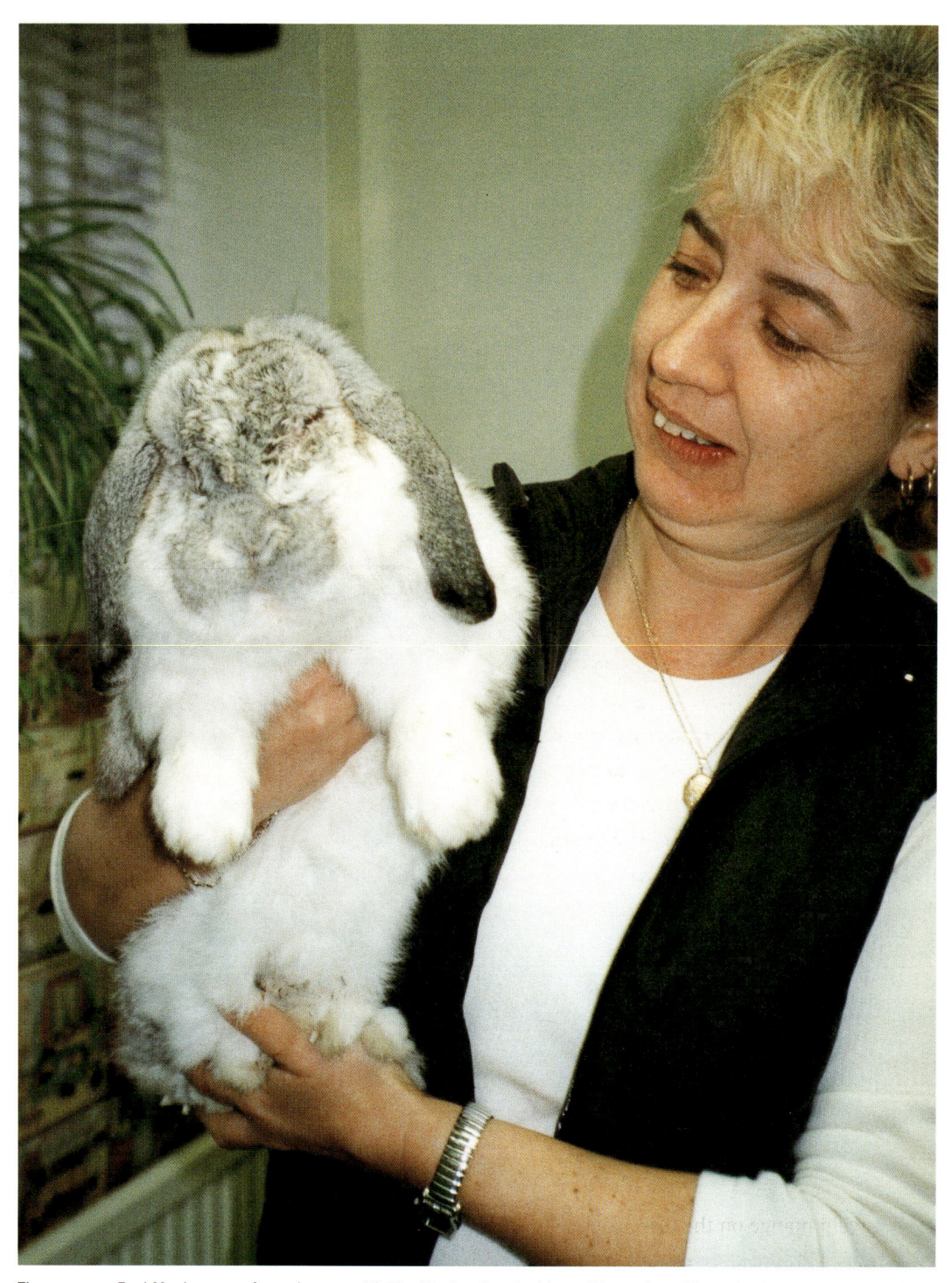

The gorgeous Fred Manley poses for a close-up with Mrs Manley. Despite his terrible teeth problems, Fred was always cheerful.

General anaesthesia can be risky for rabbits; they seem to respond badly to the stress of it. I always worry about the risk with rabbits and always feel a little depressed when I have to give them a general anaesthetic – I would hate to have to make that awful phone call if the worst should happen. However, you have to weigh the risks against the advantages and, after discussing the pros and cons at length, we decided to book a date for Fred.

The day duly arrived and poor old Fred was brought into the surgery. It took me a long time to extract the first incisor, with great care. It is so important to do it properly, because they can break off during the procedure and then they would grow back again later. Finally, after a lot of sweating and, I admit, swearing, I pulled out a long, curved tooth. It was amazing to see how little of a rabbit's incisor is actually visible above the gum: it is only about one-fifth of the whole tooth, and the rest is the curved root.

We could only extract two teeth this time, because the other two incisors had been broken off. Fred woke up after his anaesthetic and was fine; he soon went home to chew some more garden plants. Three weeks later he came back to have the last two extracted. My worry was that the infection at one of the roots was now affecting his jaw bone, but what else could we try? There was another three weeks with intensive antibiotic treatment and a change of diet to see if we could improve his bones.

> **Trude's helping hand**
>
> *Facts about rabbits' teeth*
>
> - Rabbits' teeth grow continuously and are open-rooted. Rabbits need to chew to keep their teeth in trim and wear them down.
> - A rabbit's incisor teeth can grow at the rate of 2 cm a month.

A month later we could see the improvement. For those of you who might wonder how a rabbit can manage without front teeth, the answer is that it does. It uses the cheek teeth more but can still eat the same pelleted food.

The last time I saw Fred he was fine but he still had problems with his tear ducts and his eyes. Unfortunately this seems to be a chronic problem and we are keeping it under control with medication. Teeth problems and tear ducts can be linked – if the teeth are poor and the bone is soft to the roots it will impinge on the tear ducts blocking them. Also infection from teeth roots will spread to tear ducts. Chronic thickening of ducts happens when infection has been around for a long time.

What I admire most about Fred is that he always seems to be so happy, despite his troubles. He is so lively that the last time I saw him Mrs Manley was considering giving him away, because he took up so much time and she had several other rabbits and guinea pigs to look after. For a while I considered taking him on myself, but my asthmatic sister said she would never be able to visit me if I did. So I decided against it. Anyway if he went I am sure Fred would find a lovely home – but, knowing the Manleys, I am willing to bet that they will keep him anyway.

As Fred's story shows, rabbits' teeth grow continuously and they need to wear them down on something all the time. Otherwise the teeth grow so much that they need to be cut or extracted. Rabbits also need a certain amount of fibre and calcium in the diet. If they are given the wrong type of food, especially with inadequate calcium, they develop soft skulls and may have root and other tooth problems as a result. So the content of the food is important, as is keeping an eye on their teeth and seeing that they are eating properly. The most common early symptoms in a rabbit with bad teeth are that the animal is off its food and that there is wetness under the chin from drooling. Spikes on the cheek teeth cause ulcers on the inside of cheek and tongue causing pain and anorexia.

Chinchillas, like rabbits, can have abnormally formed jaws and skulls which cause abnormal growth of the teeth. They get what people call 'slobbers' when their molars and incisors are overgrown – they are always drooling, and the poor little things have constantly damp fur on their chin, front paws and chest. It is important that chinchilla teeth are regularly rasped and cleaned if they are deformed.

Gerbils, too, can get overgrown teeth if they don't have enough chewy food, and it is the same with hamsters, which can be given pieces of wood or biscuit to chomp on. Chipmunks' incisors get too long if they are given too much soft food; given a proper diet you rarely have any health problems with them. Again, they need to chew on something, preferably twigs and nuts, to keep their teeth in good order.

And did you know that lizards have teeth? Snakes do, of course (think fangs), and both groups can get mouth rot, which starts as a gum infection and if not treated can spread into the jawbone and down the throat as well.

Diet

It is quite surprising how many of the problems in pets can be put down to the wrong diet. I have already mentioned how teeth can be affected by diet, for example, and of course the right diet is particularly important for pregnant and lactating mums, both their own sakes and for their young. In young growing animals the role of diet is crucial to their future health, but a properly balanced diet goes on playing an important part in any animal's wellbeing for the rest of its life. It's a bit like us – if we eat junk food all the time, it will show – animals need equally high quality food to look their best and be in their best health.

So the first question is: what should you feed your pet? Then comes the question of how much and how often, something that usually changes with the animal's age. All of these questions can be answered at your veterinary practice and some practices have nurses with special expertise in nutrition.

Some species are carnivores; they basically eat meat. Some are vegetarian; and some are omnivores, which means they eat quite a wide range of food, including both meat and plants. Worryingly, especially with 'exotic' pets, some owners have no idea whether their animals are carnivores or vegetarians. If your pet is more exotic than just a dog or cat, it is particularly important that you find out exactly what its real dietary needs are before you acquire it. For example, it might need to be fed 'pinkies' (baby rodents) or day-old chicks, and if you cannot find a regular supply of these, or cannot face the thought of giving them to your pet, then you should not have such a pet in the first place!

'Meat' can mean anything from minced beef and fish to earthworms, snails and insects – anything of animal origin. The problem for the owner of a truly carnivorous pet is that, in the wild, the animal might eat whole carcases, including bits of fur and bone as well as internal organs, and if you only feed the animal actual flesh it will be deprived of certain essential minerals it would find in those other parts of the carcase. Mineral and vitamin deficiencies can sometimes lead to quite serious disease.

On the other hand, it really worries me a lot and makes me quite angry when people who are vegetarians or, worse, vegans insist on giving their pets a vegetarian or vegan diet as well. You can just about get away with for a dog but never for a cat. Cats are not human beings; cats are true carnivores and cannot get all the vitamins and minerals they need unless they have meat of some kind. It is just not fair on the animal to impose your own views on it when its body systems are not designed to cope with the results.

Whatever you feed, always introduce any changes in diet or new foods gradually to avoid digestive upset. And don't forget that, for most species, fresh drinking water is an essential part of their diet as well. If

Trude's helping hand

What to feed ...

- **Dogs** are omnivores but with the emphasis on meat. As pets they are spoilt for choice; a lot of research has been done on their dietary needs and it is probably wisest to choose a commercial brand, rather than trying to make the right balance from fresh foods (which is time consuming and often more expensive). You can buy properly balanced diets as frozen, tinned, 'semi-moist' or dry food; the choice is up to you and your dog, as there are pros and cons for all of them. In general, a mature dog needs only one main meal a day but an old or sick dog would do better to have more frequent and smaller meals.

- **Cats** are true carnivores and it is even more important to get the balance of their diet right than it is for a dog. They can suffer from too much of certain vitamins as well as too little, or from vitamins coming from the wrong source (plants rather than animals). You should also be wary of feeding a cat too much of something it might have a passion for, such as liver and oily fish, and also bear in mind that milk can become indigestible to some cats once they reach maturity (though you could try goat's milk instead of cow's). As with dogs, the petfood companies have done a lot of research on cat nutrition and it is safest to choose from their 'complete diet' products rather than try to create your own from fresh foods. You can buy commercial catfood as tinned, semi-moist or dried.

- **Ferrets** are also true carnivores and can be given good commercial catfood (moist or dry) as a basic diet, or you can try the dry foods that have recently been developed specially for ferrets. But you should also give ferrets the occasional fresh dead mouse, rabbit or day-old chick.

- **Rabbits** are vegetarians; in fact by nature they are herbivores, which means they 'graze' on grass and other plants that have a high fibre content. They do like variety, so as well as a balanced diet from commercial rabbit mix or pellets, let them have access to good hay, growing grass, green weeds (dandelion leaves, groundsel, chickweed and so on), salad leaves, cabbage and a few root vegetables for gnawing.

- **Rodents** include all the other small cage mammals – rats, mice, hamsters, gerbils, guinea pigs, chinchillas, chipmunks and so on. Rats, mice and chipmunks are omnivores and opportunists – in the wild they will eat you notice that your pet is drinking a lot more than usual for no obvious reason, go and talk to your vet because this could be a sign of disease.

Obesity

At least two pets out of every three I see in my surgery, where cats and dogs are concerned, are overweight and I have to discuss weight loss and weight management with their owners. In Britain generally, almost 60%

what they can find; you can buy a basic commercial rodent mix (a combination of various grains, high-oil seeds and nuts, and pulses) and supplement it with fruit, vegetables, dog biscuits and household scraps (chipmunks also appreciate insects, eggs and even the occasional mouse). Hamsters and gerbils are basically herbivores and you can give a commercial rodent mix with a little fresh fruit and vegetables. Guinea pigs have very specific dietary requirements for vitamin C and you need to give them a commercial guinea pig mix plus plenty of good hay and fresh grass, supplemented with greenstuffs such as dandelion leaves, groundsel and vegetables. You also need to make sure that they eat up their vitamin C before it goes 'stale'. Chinchillas need grass-based chinchilla pellets and good hay plus fresh vegetables.

- **Cage birds** need plenty of variety in their food but are also very suspicious of new foods they don't recognise. You often need to mix their food well as otherwise they will simply pick out their favourite and ignore the rest, which might lead to an unbalanced diet. Some are seed-eaters (canaries, budgies etc), some are fruit-eaters,

some are insectivores (mynahs, for example, need things like live mealworms) and some feed on nectar (toucans and hummingbirds). Offer seed-eaters several different varieties of seed plus greenstuffs (chickweed, lettuce and so on), vegetables and fruit. There are plenty of commercial 'complete diet' foods available for the different species. Parrots are even fussier eaters than other birds and need to be stimulated by feeding little and often, hiding food for them and offering a good variety of at least five different kinds of seed plus three or four different kinds of vegetables and of fruit every day, with the occasional treat such as wholemeal bread, cereal or fruit cake.

- **Reptiles** vary in their dietary needs according to species and it is important to find out exactly what your particular pet requires. Snakes are carnivores and some of them need live rodents, for example; others eat earthworms and slugs, or frogs or fish. Iguanas are vegetarian but geckos and chameleons eat insects. Tortoises are vegetarians (vegetables, fruit, grass – and flowers!) but terrapins and turtles are omnivores (small fish, earthworms, baby mice and greens).

of cats and dogs are overweight. Why are British pets so fat? It may have something to do with their owners' lifestyle. For example, in my own country, Norway, the lifestyle of most people is based on walking and hiking; there is more space around and the dogs and cats are much less likely to be fat.

Obesity is related to a mismatch between calorie burning and calorie intake and people are basically giving their animals too much food and too little exercise. Dogs are probably easier to handle when it comes to overweight because they can be taken for walks and runs. Labradors, by the way, are not meant to be fat. They are meant to have a waist as slim as that of a German shepherd; they should be just slightly more stocky in build, but they are meant to have a waist!

Cats are more difficult to exercise; they are not really inclined to go for a walk on a lead like dogs (and I do not recommend it either). There are other ways of exercising a cat but perhaps it is more important to manipulate the type of food you are giving them.

People need to be a little more strict with their animals, especially when it comes to feeding. Obesity is a terrible problem in this country and it can lead to so many other dangerous conditions, such as diabetes, heart problems and hip problems. What sort of quality of life does an animal focused on food have? It should be outside enjoying pottering about, not just sitting by the fridge willing you to open it.

Animals will choose the easiest option but it is not fair on the animals and it is the owner's responsibility to keep the animal healthy and fit. In my view it is almost a case of abuse when an animal is allowed to become so fat that it cannot even walk about normally. I have seen it – and I have known so many owners fooling themselves that their pet just happens to have a small head and skinny legs, when really the animal is obese.

It is very easy to make excuses but many owners need to realise that what they are actually doing is killing their animals with kindness. They are literally shortening their pet's life span by two or three years. They simply cannot give an animal food every time it asks for it. Overweight animals suffer just as much as overweight people.

I really do believe that it is on the borderline of neglect when an owner allows their animal to become overweight. When you choose to keep a pet you take on responsibility for every aspect of its life and it is up to you to keep it as healthy as possible. It eats the food that you provide for it and so you must make sure that it is the right food and right amount. If the animal does put on a lot of weight and an unhealthy amount of fat, it is up to you to do something about it as a responsible pet owner.

Animals will eat what they are offered. They only become fussy because you give them the choice. It is the owner who is at fault. Dogs and cats are not naturally fussy with food; it is we who make them fussy. I tell my clients that they are more in control over their animals than they realise. It is just that the animals are so clever at manipulating people and playing on their owners' softer side that we go all soppy and think, 'Oh, my pet's going to love me more if I give it this piece of chocolate.' It will not love you more if you give it that piece of chocolate; that is not how animals' minds work. You are killing with kindness.

There are slimming classes for animals in most veterinary hospitals these days, and there are weight clinics where nurses will weigh your animal for free so that you can keep control of how quickly it is losing weight. It is anyway advisable to talk to your vet if you think your pet has a weight problem. Bear in mind that there are certain conditions that can make an animal put on weight, and if you feel that you are doing all the right things already but the animal keeps on ballooning out, ask for a blood sample to be taken to check for possible hormonal causes for a very slow metabolic rate or weight gain. For example, a dog with Cushing's disease will have a ravenous appetite and often develops a pot belly because the liver is enlarged. Any dramatic and sudden weight gain, or weight loss, should always be discussed with your vet, just in case it is caused by disease.

Weight loss should be gradual and controlled. Decrease the food by a third or change to food in a low-calorie diet.

Cat on the go

Sometimes what seems to be a weight problem is in fact a thyroid problem – either the thyroid gland is over-active (hyperthyroidism) or it is under-active (hypothyroidism). With dogs, an under-active thyroid gland means that they put on weight but not in the same way as with Cushing's disease. The weight goes on all over the body, even if they are eating very little food; the skin gets thick, they become very lethargic

TRUDE MOSTUE + **Pets in Practice**

> **Trude's helping hand**
>
> ### Facts about obesity
>
> - The normal weight for a cat is 3–4 kg but these days most cats seem to weigh about 5 kg, unless they are nice slim farm cats.
> - In Britain, 52% of dogs and 47% of cats are obese.
> - Obesity predisposes animals to heart and joint problems and to hormonal diseases.

and they always seem to be looking for a source of heat to sit near.

With cats, it is more likely to be an over-active thyroid gland, especially in elderly females. I remember visiting a house where there were four or five cats; one of them was incredibly skinny and she had her head stuck into a big bowl of food. As soon as she had wolfed that lot down, she stuck her head into a big tin for more and I knew straight away that this was hyperthyroidism. In this disease, all the cell metabolisms speed up and the animal burns up huge amounts of energy so it eats and eats and eats.

The trouble is, owners tend to think that if an animal is eating well and drinking well and is active, then it must be well. Typically owners bring their animals in far too late, because by then all the systems have been going at such a high rate – the heart is beating flat out,

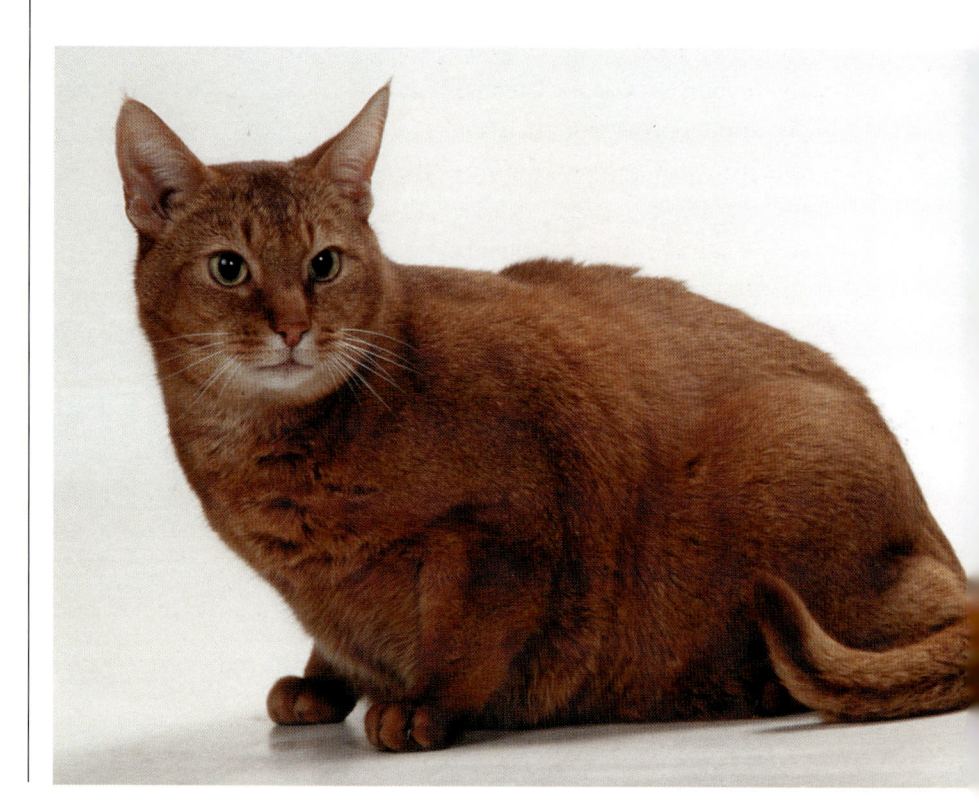

Fat cats are not always overweight because they eat too much. It may be due to a thyroid problem.

the blood goes thudding through and they end up with clots in the leg veins. Typically the owner sees their pet suddenly in agony and lame in the back legs, and then there is likely to be heart failure because the heart is working so fast. When an animal like this comes into the surgery I can see that heart rate from the other side of the room, pumping away like a mad thing, and by then it is almost too late.

Hyperthyroidism in cats means either tablets or an operation. The operation is to remove what is usually a tumour on the thyroid and it is quite expensive, so most people opt for tablets. But the tablets have to be given for the rest of the animal's life, and cats are notoriously uptight about taking pills. They don't like them at all, which means that people stop trying to dose them regularly and in no time at all the cat is a walking skeleton with that big heart beating away like crazy. This will shorten its lifespan – if left uncontrolled.

Portly pooches

The easiest way to talk about obesity in dogs is to demystify what you do. It is not that difficult: you apply the same principles as you would apply to yourself. If a dog becomes not very active and you continue to give it the same energy-rich food as you always gave when it was having plenty of exercise, of course the dog will put on weight. You have to change something and you have three main options: more exercise, lighter food or less food.

The first option is to make sure that the dog has more exercise. Where this is possible, only increase the level of exercise gently. This is especially important when an animal is very overweight, because it has to carry a lot of weight about.

If it is not possible to give the dog more exercise, you need to change the diet to one with less calorie-rich food. The main energy component in a dog's food comes from fat, so you should decrease the fat content and increase the carbohydrates and fibre. You can easily buy specially formulated foods now – you do not have to spend hours in the kitchen cooking something for the dog.

An alternative to changing the food completely is to decrease the amount of food you give. The problem with this is that the dog will let you know that it is still hungry, which puts pressure on you to give it more food. There is something with people and animals: they just cannot bear to see their pets hungry, and so they give in. Anyway, it is not nice to feel hungry, so if there is a choice between less food and different food I would definitely go for specially formulated food with a lower calorie content if your animal is getting less exercise.

The aim should be for the dog to lose weight gradually over quite a long period. Crash dieting is not healthy for animals.

Fat cats

With cats, it is more complicated: you need to concentrate more on giving them the right types of food rather than on exercise, though you can exercise cats by playing with them – perhaps with the help of little balls on elastic string to make them stretch and jump.

The problem with cats is that, once they reach a certain weight, their main focus becomes food and they do not even bother to go out any more. Of course, the less they move around, the more focused they become on food and the fatter they become; and the fatter they become, the less they want to move around, because it is too tiring. It becomes a vicious circle.

Very often, when I suggest changing a cat's diet to a lighter food, the owner tells me that the cat will not eat it. Well, cats are not stupid; they will not starve themselves to death and they will eat it eventually. I firmly believe you should be quite strict on this. Of course a cat will turn up its nose at a food that is different and will decide not to like it, given the choice. Yet in the wild cats would eat whatever they managed to catch; they would not stop to think, 'Well, that mouse looks less tasty than the other so I am not going to eat it.'

A cat will eat what it is offered but owners are sometimes too soft; they panic and rush off to buy a different food straight away. Cats are clever and they think, 'Aha! Last time I turned my nose up at this food, there was a different one on the table the very next day! So I'll do that again.'

For my weekly newspaper column in Scotland I often get people saying that their cat wakes them up in the night demanding food. And then they get up and give it food! So of course the cat knows exactly which button to press and will do it again and again. All the owner really needs to do is say no.

Beefy bunnies

The problem of obesity is now spreading to pet rabbits as well, especially when they do not have enough space to exercise and run around. I often see rabbits that are so overweight they cannot even reach around to clean their back ends, and if they are out on grass in the summer they get diarrhoea and the flies come along and suddenly they have maggots from fly-strike because they are too fat to turn and clean themselves properly. The flies lay their eggs in the mucky bottoms and the larvae will burrow into the skin, which is pretty disgusting. One problem is that fly-strike can be quite sneaky: the rabbit gradually becomes off-colour and people 'suddenly' find maggots, though actually they will have been there for some time – which is why it is so important to check your rabbit regularly in summer and to keep its back end clean. It might even be worth shaving off some of the hair to prevent flystrike. By the time you realise your rabbit is ill, there is probably only a 50:50 chance of survival so you really must take the problem seriously and do all you can to prevent it in the first place, or to treat it in the very early stages.

The best way of helping a rabbit to lose excess weight is to increase its exercise, rather than to decrease the amount of food.

Elvis the iguana

When I worked at Longleat, we had a family of iguanas named after members of the Presley family. The male, Elvis, was so named for very good reason: he had nutritional osteoporosis and deformed jaws that gave him a real Elvis curl of the lip and snarl!

Iguanas are amazing animals and stunning to look at, but people who buy them when they are about 10 centimetres long do not appreciate that they will grow to a metre or more, which means they will need a whole room to themselves to thrash about in. They can also become quite aggressive under stress and they do have knife-sharp claws (as I know to my cost). They are definitely not pets for children.

Iguanas are of course reptiles. About 80% of the veterinary problems seen in reptiles are related to the wrong nutrition or to poor husbandry. They are kept at the wrong temperature or wrong humidity, for example, so that they have difficulty in shedding their skins, or they are kept alone and become unhappy. I also quite often see egg-bound snakes. None of the reptiles are really pets for children, who don't have the time, knowledge and sustained interest to look after them properly.

Many pet reptiles have calcium deficiency, which leads to brittle bones and bone breakages, and when I talk to the owner I soon discover that the animal has been fed the wrong diet. Sometimes it is so bad that the bones do not show up at all on the X-ray. Often people have taken over a reptile from a friend and really have no idea about its true needs. It is a lack of commitment on their part, because plenty of information is available – even more so now with the internet. There really is no excuse for pleading ignorance, and perhaps if it was compulsory for owners to go on a course before any pet shop would sell them a reptile, it would save everyone a lot of trouble and make for a lot more happiness among the reptiles themselves. Most of them are not native to Britain anyway and so their needs are bound to be special.

Quite a few reptiles are kept in collections by adults, rather than being kept as pets by children. Many of them go to specialists when the reptiles are unwell.

Tortoises, which have become so valuable in recent years because of import restrictions, can live for many, many years (longer than humans) but they are increasingly rare on their native Mediterranean hillsides. They require very particular conditions for hibernation in winter and are not as easy to look after as some people think. At Longleat we had about 50 of them and used a big old refrigerator for hibernation, stacking them in boxes inside it. The ideal temperature for hibernation of Mediterranean tortoises is about 4°C. Tortoises also need their beaks trimmed – definitely a job for the specialist.

Tortoises are in the group known as chelonians; terrapins are in the same group and both species often suffer from dietary calcium deficiency, especially when they are young, leading to very soft shells. Terrapins, unlike tortoises, feed in water and spend quite a lot of time in it. They can be really quite vicious and, again, they are often bought rather thoughtlessly when they are tiny without people realising how much they will grow. The awful thing is that people then go and dump them in a local pond, which is a bit unfair on the terrapin and even more unfair on other creatures in the pond, as terrapins eat fish, tadpoles, water snails, molluscs and other meaty goodies in there.

Lumps and bumps

It is always worrying for an owner to find a lump on their pet – they immediately think of cancer but not all lumps are cancerous. Very often a lump is a tick, or an abscess, or something else much less nasty than cancer. Lots of different species get assorted lumps and bumps and it is always worth having them checked out by the vet to put your mind at rest, though the outcome is not always a happy one.

With a lump, it is important to be able to describe it in everyday terms, when you are telling your vet about how much it has grown over a certain period. For example, is it like an apple, or is it more a walnut or a grape?

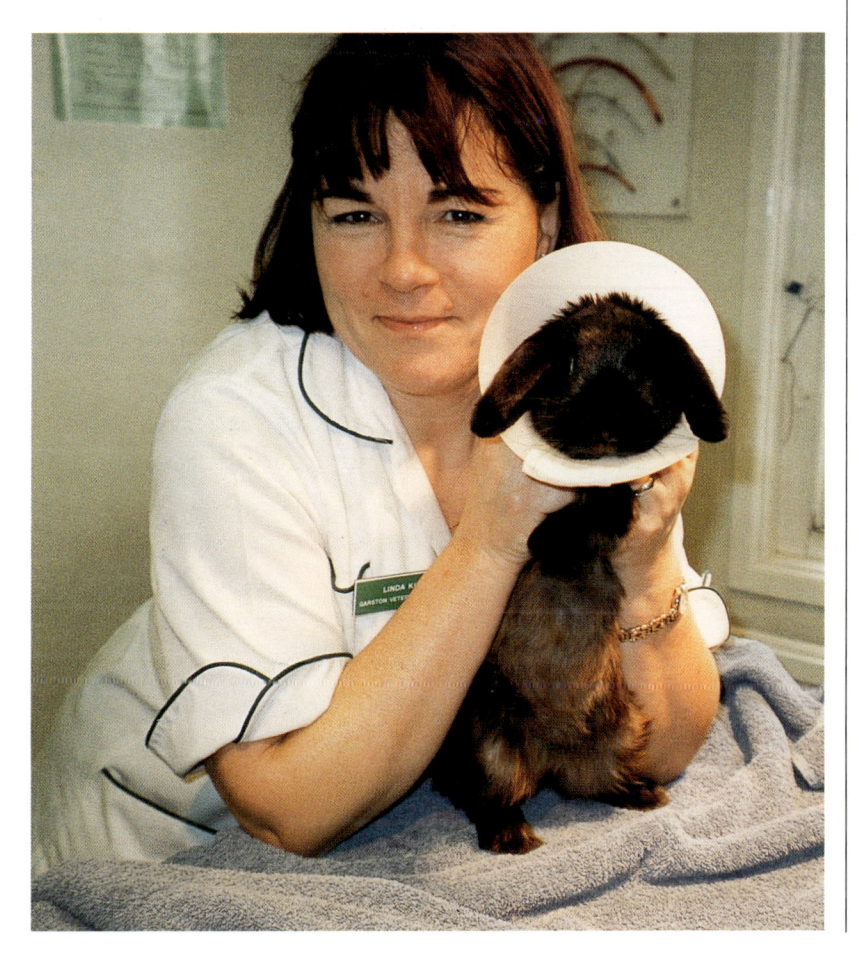

My friend Linda King poses with Desmond Bolster, my favourite rabbit.

Desmond's lumps

Desmond Bolster was a little black lop-eared rabbit and when he first came to see me at about three months old he had a nasty abscess on his back; it was almost bigger than he was. Rabbit abscesses can be very awkward to deal with: they are usually more severe than in other animals and are difficult to get rid of as they have a habit of coming back time and time again.

Desmond was a wonderful character. He arrived in a bucket, and would always come in his bucket on the many occasions he had to return to the surgery after that first visit. The abscess was big and I thought it might be a tumour and so I had to anaesthetise him to clean it out. It turned out not to be a tumour after all and he came safely through the anaesthetic, which is always a worry with rabbits. They are such nervous animals, and they frighten so easily. So I was happy to bring him through that first operation successfully and I hoped that would be it.

When I was talking to the owner, she told me that it might have been caused in the first place by a bite from the guinea pig he lived with, but I still do not know if that was it. I only knew that his abscess was a traumatic reaction in the skin and, as with other rabbit abscesses, I had cleaned it out and hoped for the best. But, as with so many rabbits, he came back two weeks later because it had filled up again – it seemed almost like a whole chain of abscesses on his back.

For the next two months, Desmond was back and forth to the surgery for treatment with antibiotics and still he did not seem to mind whether he was on my table or at home on the grass. In he would come in his bucket, and in the waiting-room he was king: I'd sometimes hear a Rottweiler confronting Desmond thumping in his bucket but Desmond would always outstare any dog and it would be the Rottweiler that would back off, whimpering. Then Desmond would sit on my table washing himself, quite unconcerned about me and the nurses or even the television camera crew. After a while he would growl and stamp his feet at me, just to show who was the boss here, and would rip the towel to shreds to prove his point. He was getting a bit fed up with his abscesses, a bit fed up with his owner chasing him every day to give him his antibiotic and deal with his back, and a bit fed up with me chasing him too. He was an all-action rabbit!

After two months of this I decided I needed to do quite radical surgery to cut out the whole abscess. It was a major operation and I was worried at the thought of another anaesthetic for him. It took about an hour and a half and I managed to remove it encapsulated; there were about three capsules, leaving him with a really long wound. That, I thought, really must be it this time and he recovered really well from the operation and from the anaesthetic.

Two weeks later he came back to have his stitches out, which of course he had tried to do for himself, and he seemed fine. With a sigh of relief, I sent him home to be happy ever after in his hutch.

In March, about four or five months after his first visit, Desmond's owner rang me up in tears. The abscess was back and she was ready to give up – she could not face more of the endless surgery visits. It was not the money; she would happily pay if I could cure him once and for all. He came in again in his bucket, all bright and busy; he sat on the table and washed himself as usual, and got annoyed with me as usual, and I had to confirm that the abscess was back. If we left it there, he would die. If we operated again, I could not guarantee to the owner that it would not come back.

We agreed to put him to sleep and I was truly devastated – to give up on a rabbit just because of an abscess. It was so hard: he was such a character and he seemed so happy with life on the whole, and as a vet I hate to give up. But I could not promise the owner, who had become a good friend, that it would all be okay after a third operation; I could not put her through all that again. It reminded me that I cannot cure everything and that rabbit abcesses can be incredibly persistent.

It also reminded me that some people (not Mrs Bolster though) look on vets as car mechanics. You treat an animal; say, you drain a cyst, but it comes back again and sometimes I have had quite bad confrontations with owners who are angry that the operation has not cured the problem. But animals are not cars, they do not have mechanical parts; living tissue is unpredictable and much more complicated than metal. Not everything can be mended and sometimes enough is enough. It is frustrating for me and frustrating for the owners, but there it is.

With Desmond, we could do no more for him. In the wild, he would have died long before. Happily, his owner has another little bunny now – but if I find it is living with that guinea pig, I shall scream!

Ratty's bumps

It is not only rabbits that have lumps. Rats often have them as well; they are very prone to skin tumours and I usually see a rat with lumps at least once a week. Most rat owners are aware of this tendency and monitor the lumps to see how much they grow. The faster they grow, the more likely it is that they are malignant, though not necessarily – in fact many rats live quite happily with their lumps and as long as they are not bothered by them that is fine. We remove quite a few lumps but they do often come back again and, as with Desmond, the anaesthetic is always a risk and you reach a point where it is no longer ethical to subject them to another operation. Sometimes the tumours spread to the chest and other systems and that is really time to call it a day.

A nice little rat came in when she was about four years old, which is a good age for a rat, though I have seen some that lived to five or six. (Three would be old for a hamster.) She had a really big and aggressive lump and the owner insisted that I should remove it. Well, some lumps shell out easily and you simply close the wound, but this one was attached to the lymphatic system and I knew it would come back. And with a rat they do not have a lot of blood anyway, so they cannot afford to lose much of it.

Anyway, the owner was insistent and so I removed the lump. She was fine for a while afterwards but then it all came back somewhere else on her body and I felt she had been through enough last time. The owner agreed, and we put the little rat to sleep.

Trude's helping hand

The drawbacks of animals getting older

- The most common problem in an ageing animal is its teeth, and it is during middle age that poor dental hygiene really begins to show, especially if (in the case of dogs) they do not chew on sticks and bones.
- There might be heart problems, usually as a result of overweight.
- Liver or kidney problems might develop.
- Diabetes is quite common at this age, particularly again with overweight animals, and so any sign of increased thirst and decreased appetite should be checked out.
- Problems with hips and arthritic joints are common in elderly pets, as with elderly people. Again, if the pet is overweight these problems will be worse than they have to be.

Rats are wonderful pets, though some people do not like them because of their tails and because of folk memories of the plague and so on. They are very intelligent and friendly; they hardly ever bite and seem to love human company, and they are not nocturnal animals like hamsters. They are easy to train, too, and I think they make better pets for children than hamsters.

Growing old

As an animal grows older, naturally you will need to keep a more careful eye on potential problems connected with ageing. It is worth bringing them in to see the vet for six-monthly check-ups so that anything which might be going wrong can be treated sooner rather than later.

In terms of years, 'old age' is very different between cats and dogs. I would not consider a cat to be even middle-aged before it is around 10 years old and many live twice as long as that. With dogs it really depends on the breed. The smaller breeds seem to live for longer than the larger breeds so they reach middle age and old age later in life. For example, most poodles easily reach the age of 15, but 12 is old for a labrador and the average lifespan of a Great Dane is only about nine years.

So an average labrador-size dog will start to approach middle age when it is about eight years old and this is when the first signs of ageing will begin to appear.

Rats, like rabbits, are very prone to skin tumours which commonly take the form of harmless bumps.

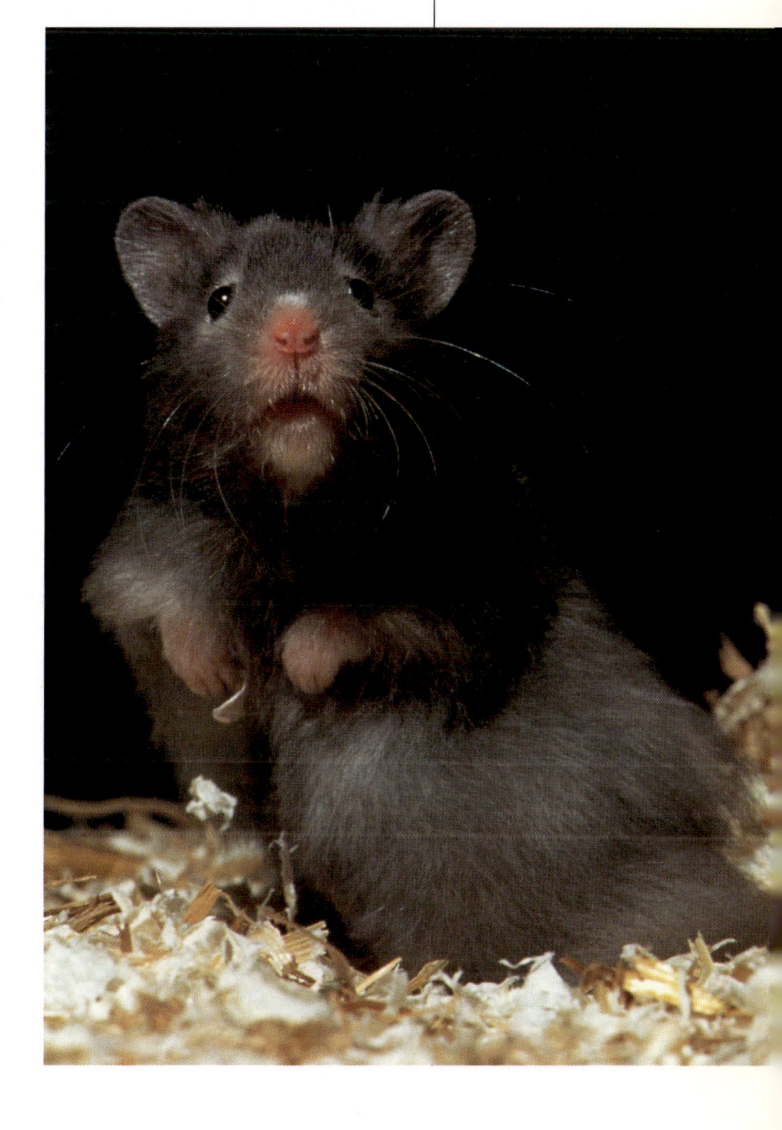

A good old age

A healthy, active lifestyle and appropriate weight are so important. I often notice that the patients who have been a normal weight all their life look so much better when they are reaching old age, and they last for longer as well because they are healthier.

Old age is inevitable but sometimes owners do not seem to appreciate that pets get old, just like people do. They find it difficult to accept that a 12-year-old labrador, which is really the equivalent of an 85-year-old human being, does not want to jump the fences any more. I would not expect that from my grandad, so why on earth would you expect that from a dog? Perhaps because animals do not always *look* old, in the way that we humans do, we tend to have greater expectations of them, but you should treat them as old people: you should accept that they have a slower pace of life, that they walk more slowly and run more slowly. You need to find a lifestyle that keeps them exercising, but at a slower pace.

As with old people, old animals' immune systems do not seem to cope well with challenges any more, and so you need to keep an eye on their gums, and keep an eye on the coat to check for fleas and other parasites. You also need to keep an eye on the claws – it is amazing how many people let their pets' claws grow very long, even growing into their pads.

Finally, there will probably come a time when you have to make that most heart-breaking decision of all, when your ageing pet's quality of life is no longer good and you, as its owner, have the responsibility for calling it a day and asking your vet to put it to sleep.

Saying goodbye

Putting an animal to sleep is one of the most important things we do in veterinary practice, which may sound bizarre. I never realised that was going to be the case when I graduated, though of course I knew it would be a big part of what we do and it is a situation we have to be able to handle well.

The most worrying part of euthanasia is knowing that if you do not do it well and if you do not treat the owners sensitively or appropriately, you are going to be remembered for it and people will not come back to you. It is a known fact that the most important memory people have of a veterinary surgeon concerns the euthanasia of a particular animal.

For most people, pets are members of the family. Even if it is a gerbil, its loss can be emotionally serious for a child. People become incredibly attached to everything from small rodents up to horses, and the animal becomes a part of the family. It is very important for veterinary surgeons to understand that.

Because you are tired and you work a lot and you see a lot of animals coming through your surgery door, it is very easy to become a little cynical and lose the emotional involvement. I do not mean that vets should cry or lose their professional attitude, but it is really important to hold on to your empathy with the owners when you are dealing with euthanasia.

Very often people come into my surgery and I know what they want me to do without them telling me. Sometimes, if they bring in a very sick animal, they really want me to make the decision for them, but at the same time they want to be ready for it. You should never rush anyone into a decision about euthanasia but at the same time you should never let anyone hold on to an animal just because it hurts to let it go.

Over-attachment to the animal is probably one of the main problems with the way people keep pets in today's society. It is so hard to let something go when you love it a lot, and it is an awful decision to make because people feel as if they are killing a member of the family. That decision is very hard to make, and this is something that we as veterinary surgeons should understand. An old dog is not just an old animal for a family that has had it for 12 or 13 years. Even worse, a cat someone has had for 21 years is not just a grumpy old cat. It is a family member. The tricky part is to find out if people are ready for the decision and to guide them into the decision gently but also in an understanding way so that they do not have this very strong guilt about their decision.

I have often talked to people about comparing euthanasia of pets with what happens in human medicine. Many people, after they have decided on euthanasia for their pet and we have done it, feel hugely relieved and they often say that the same option should be available for humans. They feel that no animal should be allowed to suffer in the way that a lot of human beings suffer in hospital or people with terminal cancer.

Euthanasia is a dark aspect of my job but it is one of the most important things you do in practice. People will remember you for it. The times when you get chocolate and cards, the times when people thank you, are after you have put their animals to sleep. It might seem surprising at first but if you have had an animal yourself you realise how grateful you are when someone handles the situation in a sensitive way and appreciates the emotional involvement with an animal and how much it can mean to someone.

A lonely old man

One day I was called out by an old man in his 80s. He had called out other vets before to have his dog put to sleep (I was the third, I think) but I did not know that at the time. I turned up at his house

Trude's helping hand

Grieving

It is entirely natural and healthy to grieve for the loss of a pet and it helps to know that your reactions are not unusual. Many people go through the same recognised stages of grief for a pet as they might for another person, though some of these stages may last only briefly and some may run into each other.

1. **Shock and disbelief** at what has happened or that euthanasia is the only course that makes sense. Even worse is if your pet has died suddenly after an accident, especially a young animal, and it seems so unfair. This sense of shock will usually last for less than a day.

2. **Anger and guilt** are common emotions. You might feel guilty that your pet has died, and it is very easy to seek to blame someone else for it and so you get angry. The guilt (and the anger) are usually misplaced. Some people feel guilty that they didn't see how ill their pet was soon enough, didn't seek advice earlier, or couldn't afford more treatment, when they really should not blame themselves at all.

3. **Depression** is something worse than the sadness we all feel when a beloved animal dies. With depression you cannot eat properly, you cannot sleep, you generally lose interest in your daily life and you might find yourself weeping for no real reason. Most people do not suffer from this type of depression but, if you do, have a chat with your vet or the veterinary nurse for help. They will understand.

4. **Acceptance** is when you are beginning to recover from the loss of your pet and can talk about it without getting too upset. It helps if you can remember the good times you had together, and some people find comfort in commemorating their pet in some way – perhaps by sponsoring an animal in a rescue centre.

TRUDE MOSTUE + **Pets in Practice**

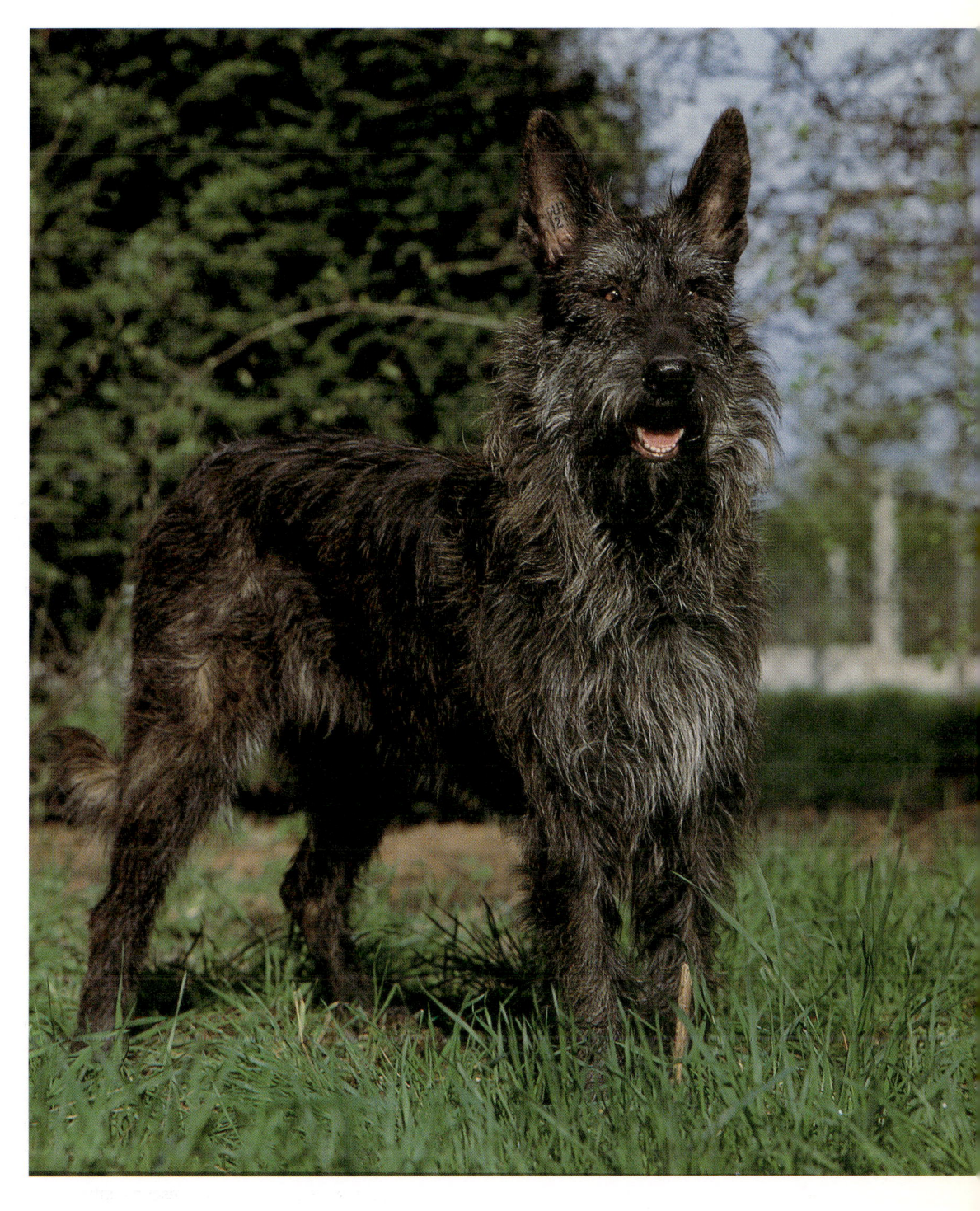

An old dog can be a great comfort to an old person. But like its owner it is essential that the animal is well looked after.

with my nurse and found this little dog lying in its basket in a corner of the kitchen. The dog was desperately thin, very old, and not with it at all. Many old animals develop senile dementia and this seemed to be quite a typical case. The dog just slept in its basket all day long. Its quality of life was very poor; it was incontinent, it had kidney failure – you name it, this poor dog had it. It had obviously come to the end of its days and was just waiting for someone to release it from a life it could no longer enjoy.

It is quite important to remember, in these situations, that in the wild an animal like this would have died long ago, unable to defend itself from predators. Instead, we have to make the decision for that animal.

When I walked into the kitchen I soon realised that this poor old man simply did not want to let his dog go; he could not bear to lose it. I think that, deep down, he knew that he had to release it but it was his only companion in life. He had no family, he had no wife, he had no children; he only had this dog, which had lived with him for about 16 years.

I was quite a recent graduate at that time and it was hard to push the issue. Obviously the dog needed to be put to sleep but the old man needed a companion and some sort of reassurance that he was not going to be alone after the dog had gone, that he would have other friends and could even have another dog. The problem with old people, though, is when they reach the age at which it is difficult for them to get another dog. They cannot take on a puppy because they know that they will probably not outlive the puppy and because they do not think it is fair for a young animal to have someone who cannot walk a lot and cannot exercise them enough. In fact, even the rescue centres will refuse to allow an old person to have one of their animals because they anticipate that the owner will die before the pet does.

The old man was distraught about it but in the end I did euthanase the little old dog. It was deeply traumatic: he was crying his eyes out, sitting on a chair with tears streaming down his face, and it was heart-breaking to watch an old man crying alone in his tiny flat, with no pictures of any relatives to keep him company. 'I have no one. I have no one,' he kept saying as he sobbed his heart out. So I stayed with him for a long while afterwards, just talking to him. It seemed to help.

When I left, I suggested that he should come and see me in the surgery if he wanted to talk, and he did just that a while later. We discussed the possibility of another dog for him and, despite what the rescue centres usually say, I know that there are quite a few old dogs needing homes. So I found an old dog for the old man. He brought it in soon after for its vaccinations and he was a different person: it was as if the sun was shining from his face.

Farewell to Jenny

Dealing with euthanasia is even sadder when I know that the animal has been through a lot. This was the case with a little Jack Russell terrier called Jenny.

Jenny hated me. She hated all vets and she hated being handled by anybody except her owners. She had had enough of us.

She was about 16 and was approaching her 'end days'. She had become incontinent and was drinking excessively. I tried to find out why. She was still very bright mentally and her owners felt it was worth trying to sort out the drinking and incontinence even though, at her age, there were plenty of other things wrong. Because she was wetting all over the house, they had confined her to the conservatory, where she had very little contact with the rest of the family, and they were beginning to feel that this was unfair on her. Something needed to be done, but they did not want to spend too much time or money on it. If I found a problem that could easily be fixed, then we would go ahead with whatever I recommended.

I took a look at her, I took blood samples and so on but in due course they decided to give up further investigations and just wait and see for a while. One day I had a message from them asking me to come out and put her to sleep, but before I could do so there was another message cancelling the first one. They were finding it very hard to make that final decision, as she was still quite bright, still running about, still sniffing your leg and so on. It was just that she had to be confined to the conservatory and not given the freedom of the house any more, which is not a great life. I can understand their difficulty. If you cannot really live with a dog any more and she spends much of her time sleeping anyway, what is her quality of life? In the end, quality of life is what it is all about.

TRUDE MOSTUE **+ Pets in Practice**

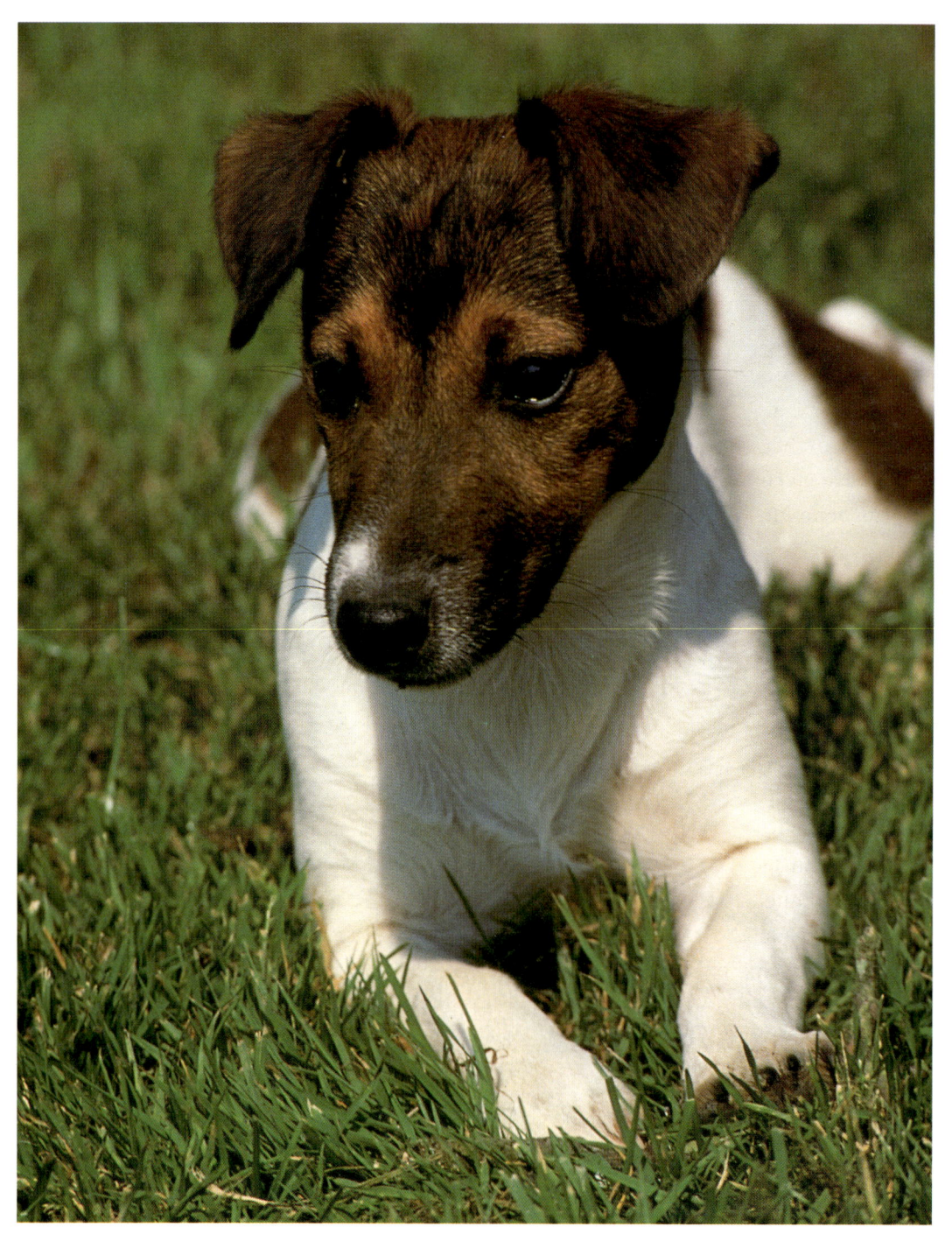

Although putting your pet to sleep seems ghastly, if it is done at the right time and for the right reasons, it will probably be the right solution.

Yet again I was called out and I realised that this time they had made their decision so I went out to the house to put her to sleep. When it comes to euthanasia I always suggest to my closest clients that I come out to them and do it at home, so that neither they nor the animal have the distress of being at the surgery.

At the house there was a really good atmosphere, which sounds strange but that is how it was. The owners were very sad, of course, but by now they were fully prepared for what was to come; they had accepted that the time was right and it had been quite easy to make the decision.

Knowing how Jenny hated being handled by vets, and that she would struggle and become really angry with me, I decided it was best to sedate her while she was in her owner's arms. Normally I would have given her a direct intravenous overdose or anaesthetic but with Jenny it was not appropriate. So I gave her a good dose of sedative in a simple subcutaneous injection while her owner held her. Then Jenny ran around the conservatory for a while before going to her basket and falling asleep. I gave her the final injection while she was unconscious.

Everything about Jenny's ending seemed to be right. The owners were ready for it; Jenny was at home, she was held by her owners, she simply went to sleep in her own basket and that was that. I think all of us felt that we did the right thing. The owners appreciated that I had taken their feelings seriously, and they realised they needed to make the decision on Jenny's behalf without being selfish. It was her quality of life that counted in the end.

Sometimes old animals are like old people: you can't expect the whole world from them and they are just tired of living. They may or may not be in pain – it is easier, perhaps, to make the decision if they are in pain, but it is just as important to do so when they are not, when they are simply at the end of their time and have no quality of life. The more attached you are to an animal, the more difficult the decision becomes to let them go, but you need to be fair to them. You need to make the decision for them and for their sake, not for your own.

INDEX

A

abscesses 15, 61, 129, 130–131
acids 42
adder bites 52, 53
aggression 8–15, 62
   cats 24–25
   dogs 8–15, 25
   fear 10, 25
   ferrets 62
   rabbits 26
alkalis 42
alpha dogs 10–12
amphibians 72
anaemia 88, 101–102, 111
anaesthetic risk 60, 61–62
   rabbits 115, 117, 130
   rats 132
anti-freeze 37, 41
arsenic 42
arthritis 132
attention seeking 20–21

B

Babesia 111
barbiturates 42
barking 20–23
behavioural problems 7–33
birds 72
   choosing 75
   diet 121
   emergencies 52
   heatstroke 36
   housing 29
   mites 109
   poisoning 40–41
   worms 101
birth 64–65, 68–69
bleach 41
bleeding 47–48
bloat 51, 52
British dog ticks 111
budgies 29, 33, 72, 109, 121
burns 52, 53

C

cages 28–29
calcium deficiency 128
canaries 109, 121
cancer 58–59, 129
castor-bean tick 111
cat 'flu 92, 94
cats
   abscesses 15

aggression 24–25
birth 65, 68–69
breeds 70
and children 23–24
choosing 74
diet 119–120
emergencies 52
FeLV 88, 91–92, 94
FIP 89–91
FIV 87–89, 92
fleas 101–105
health checks 108
neutering 24, 60–61
obesity 121–123, 124, 126
old age 133
panting 36
Paracetamol 39
pregnancy 64, 68
ringworm 109
road traffic accidents 43–47
separation anxiety 18–20
spraying 18, 19, 21, 23–24, 60
teeth problems 113–115
thyroid problems 124–125
ticks 110, 111
vaccinations 91–92, 93–94
worms 98–100, 101
children 23–24
chinchillas 29, 31, 70, 101
   diet 120, 121
   fur chewing 31, 109
   fur slip 31, 110
   ringworm 109
   teeth problems 113, 118
chipmunks 29, 31–32
   diet 118, 120–121
   teeth 118
chlamydia 33, 92, 94
choking 52
cockatiels 29, 32, 33
Cushing's disease 123

D

demulcents 40, 42
destructive behaviour 17–18, 27
diabetes 132
diarrhoea 52
diet 113–114, 119–129
   birds 121
   cats 119–120
   chinchillas 120, 121
   chipmunks 118, 120–121
   dogs 119, 120
   ferrets 120

gerbils 120–121
guinea pigs 120, 121
hamsters 120–121
mice 120–121
obesity 122–127
rabbits 115, 117, 118, 120
rats 120–121
reptiles 121, 128–129
docking 76–78
dogs
   aggression 8–15, 25
   barking 20–23
   birth 64–65, 68–69
   bleeding 47–48
   breed problems 64–65, 67, 76, 78–81
   breeds 65–70
   choosing 72–74
   Cushing's disease 123
   destructive behaviour 17–18
   diet 119, 120
   docking 76–78
   emergencies 52
   fits 36–37, 38
   fleas 103–105
   health checks 108
   heatstroke 36
   hypothyroidism 123–124
   neutering 57–59
   obesity 20, 121–123, 124, 125–126
   old age 133–134
   parvovirus 85–86, 94
   paw injuries 48–49
   poisoning 36–37
   pregnancy 64, 68
   ringworm 109
   separation anxiety 17–18
   sexual behaviour 56–57
   stings 53
   teeth problems 113–115
   temperament 81
   ticks 111
   toilet training 15–16, 17
   toy injuries 49
   vaccinations 55–56, 74, 87, 92, 93–94
   working 15–17, 48, 67, 80
   worms 74, 99
dominance 9–15
dystocia 64–65

E

elderly pets 132, 133–141

emergencies 35–53
emetics 40, 42
epilepsy 37–38
euthanasia 134–141
eyes
   inflammation 52
   prolapsed 52

F

fear aggression 10, 25
feather-plucking 32–33
feline immuno-deficiency virus (FIV) 87–89, 92
feline infectious peritonitis (FIP) 89–91
feline leukaemia virus (FeLV) 88, 91–92, 94
FeLV see feline leukaemia virus
ferrets 61–63
   aggression 62
   diet 120
   fleas 107
   heatstroke 36
   housing 28
   mites 108
   ticks 111
   types 72
   vaccinations 93, 94
fighting 12–13, 15, 61
finances 81
FIP see feline infectious peritonitis
first aid 53
fish 36, 72
fits 28–29, 36–39, 40, 42, 52
FIV see feline immuno-deficiency virus
flea dermatitis 103
fleas 83, 99, 100, 101–107
fly-strike 127
foot rot 108
fur slip 31, 110

G

gas/fumes poisoning 40–41, 42
gastric dilatation/volvulus syndrome 51
gerbils 27–29
   diet 120–121
   fits 28–29
   housing 28
   mites 109
   ringworm 109
   tapeworm 101
   teeth 118
grief 136

INDEX

guinea pigs 52
  breeds 70–71
  diet 120, 121
  handling 29–30
  housing 28–29
  mites 109
  ringworm 109

H

halitosis 52
hamsters 30–31, 71, 93
  diet 120–121
  emergencies 52
  housing 28
  mites 109
  ringworm 109
  tapeworm 101
  teeth 118
heart
  problems 132
  rate 124–125
heatstroke 36, 52
hedgehog ticks 111
herbicides 41, 42
hip dysplasia 74, 78–79
house training 15–16, 17
housing 28–29
hyperthyroidism 123–125
hypothyroidism 123–124

I

iguanas 121, 127
insecurity 15–16, 17–20

L

lead poisoning 41, 42
lice 109
lizards 72, 109, 118
lumps 129–133
Lyme's disease 111

M

malocclusion 115
mammary tumours 58–59
mange 83, 106, 107, 109
Manx cats 70
matches 41, 42
mice 31, 72, 101
  diet 120–121
  housing 28
  ringworm 109
microchips 45, 96, 97
mites 83, 106, 107–108
moulting 33

mouth rot 118
myxomatosis 92–93, 94, 107

N

nervousness 15–16, 81
neutering 24, 26, 55, 57–63, 65
non-steroidal anti-inflammatory drugs (NSAIDs) 41

O

obesity 121–127, 132
  cats 121–123, 124, 126
  dogs 20, 121–123, 124, 125–126
  rabbits 127
organophosphates 41

P

Paracetamol 39
paralysis 79
paraquat 41
parasites 32, 83, 97–111
  fleas 83, 99, 100, 101–107
  mites 83, 106, 107–108
  ticks 83, 97, 107, 109, 110–111, 129
  worms 74, 98–101, 103
parrots 29, 32–33, 72, 75, 121
parvovirus 85–86, 94
passports 94–97
paw injuries 48–49
perfume 41
pesticides 41, 42
Pet Travel Scheme (PETS) 94–97
phenols 42
pheromones 24
phosphorus 42
pigeons 109
pneumothorax 44
poisoning 36–37, 39–42
pregnancy 64, 68
psittacosis 33
pyometra 58, 60

R

rabbits
  aggression 26
  birth 65
  breeds 71–72
  diet 115, 117, 118, 120
  fleas 107
  health checks 108
  heatstroke 36
  housing 28

  lumps 130–132
  mites 108
  neutering 26
  obesity 127
  pad injuries 49
  ringworm 109
  teeth 113, 115–118
  vaccinations 92–93, 94
  worms 101
rabies 94, 96, 97
rats 31, 37, 72
  diet 120–121
  emergencies 52
  housing 28
  lumps 132–133
  mites 109
  ringworm 109
  tapeworm 101
  tumours 132
red mite 109
reptiles 27, 72, 127–129
  choosing 74–75
  diet 121, 128–129
  housing 29
rewards 21
ringworm 109
road traffic accidents 43–47, 58, 61
rodenticides 41
roundworms 99–101

S

sarcoptic mange 106, 107
scale rot 109
separation anxiety 17–20, 32–33
septicaemia 61, 113
sexual behaviour 56–57
shampoo 41
sheep ticks 111
slug bait 36–37, 41, 42
snakes 72
  diet 121
  egg-bound 128
  mites 109
  mouth rot 118
  worms 101
socialization 8, 9, 16, 21
sprains 53
spraying 18, 19, 21, 23–24, 60
status epilepticus 38
stereotypical behaviour 27, 31
stick injuries 49
stings 52, 53
stitches 48
strains 53

strychnine 42

T

tapeworms 97, 99, 100, 101, 103
tear ducts 117–118
teeth
  brushing 114–115
  problems 113–118, 132
temperament, dogs 81
terrapins 101, 121, 128–129
territorial behaviour 10, 12, 19, 23–24, 60
thirst 52, 121
thyroid problems 123–125
ticks 83, 97, 107, 109, 110–111, 129
toilet training 15–16, 17
tortoises 101, 121, 128
Toxocara
  T. canis 99, 100
  T. cati 99, 100
toy injuries 49
training 21, 25–26
tumours
  mammary 58–59
  rabbits 130
  rats 132

U

urination frequency 52

V

vaccinations 83, 84, 92–94
  cats 91–92, 93–94
  dogs 55–56, 74, 87, 92, 93–94
  ferrets 93, 94
  rabbits 92–93, 94
  rabies 96–97
vaginal discharge 52
vegetarianism 119–120
viral haemorrhagic disease (VHD) 93, 94, 107
vomiting 40, 42, 51, 52

W

warfarin 41
weight loss/gain 51, 123, 125–127
working dogs 15–17, 48, 67, 80
worms 74, 98–101, 103

143

USEFUL ADDRESSES

Amateur Entomological Society
PO Box 8774
London SW7 5ZG

Association for the Study of Reptiles and Amphibians
PO Box 73
Banbury
Oxon OX15 8RE

Association of Pet Behaviour Counsellors
PO Box 46
Worcester
WR8 9YS
01386 751151
www.apbc.org.uk

British Houserabbit Association
PO Box 346
Newcastle upon Tyne
NE99 1FA
SAE for information on house-training your rabbit

British Veterinary Dental Association
Tan y Coed
Penlon
High Street
Bangor
LL57 1PX
01248 355674

Feline Advisory Bureau
01747 871872

The Kennel Club
1-5 Clarges Street
Piccadilly
London
W1Y 8AB
0870 606 6750
info@the-kennel-club.org.uk

National Canine Defence League
17 Wakley Street
London EC1V 7RQ
020 7837 0006
www.ncdl.org.uk

National Rabbit Aid
Bristol HQ
108 Staple Hill Road
Fishponds
Bristol BS16 5AH

Pet Bereavement Helpline
0800 0966606

RSPCA
Enquiries Service
Causeway
Horsham
West Sussex RH12 1HG
01403 264181
If requesting a leaflet, please enclose 2 first class stamps

24 hour cruelty hotline
0870 5555 999
www.rspca.org.uk

The Parrot Society UK
108b Fenlake Road
Bedford MK42 0EU
01234 358922
fax 01234 359922